Clinical Dermatology For Primary Care

ADRIAAN NEL
MB.ChB *Stellenbosch University, South Africa*
LMCC, CCFP *College of Family Physicians of Canada*
Postgraduate Diploma in Clinical Dermatology *Queen Mary University of London*

For Martini...
Author, role model, mother.

FIRST EDITION

CONTENTS

Introduction

The importance of Dermatology is often overlooked during the years spent as a medical student but the importance is soon realized once you're faced with a real life problem in your clinic. Skin disease is a very substantial portion of the average day-to-day patient population in primary care and failure to address a skin issue can cause a lot of psychological and physical distress for the patient.

This book is not as textbook for specialists or dermatology residents, but as a basic general overview of the most common conditions that students and primary care doctors will encounter on a daily basis. The goal of this book is to give easy access in electronic format to common dermatology issues and treatments for students and family physicians.

In this book we tried to group conditions with similar appearances together in order for the reader to have easy access to the right topic once he or she identified the morphology of the lesion.

Medical research, knowledge and treatments are constantly evolving. We try to give the most up to date advice in order to provide the basic treatment in the readers' clinics but all treatments and drugs should be verified with the manufacturer's recommendations on how to administer the drug and at what dose. It is the responsibility of the reader to determine the best treatment, dosage and contraindications for each patient. Neither the publisher nor the author assumes any liability for any injury or damage to persons or property arising from this publication.

Describing skin lesions

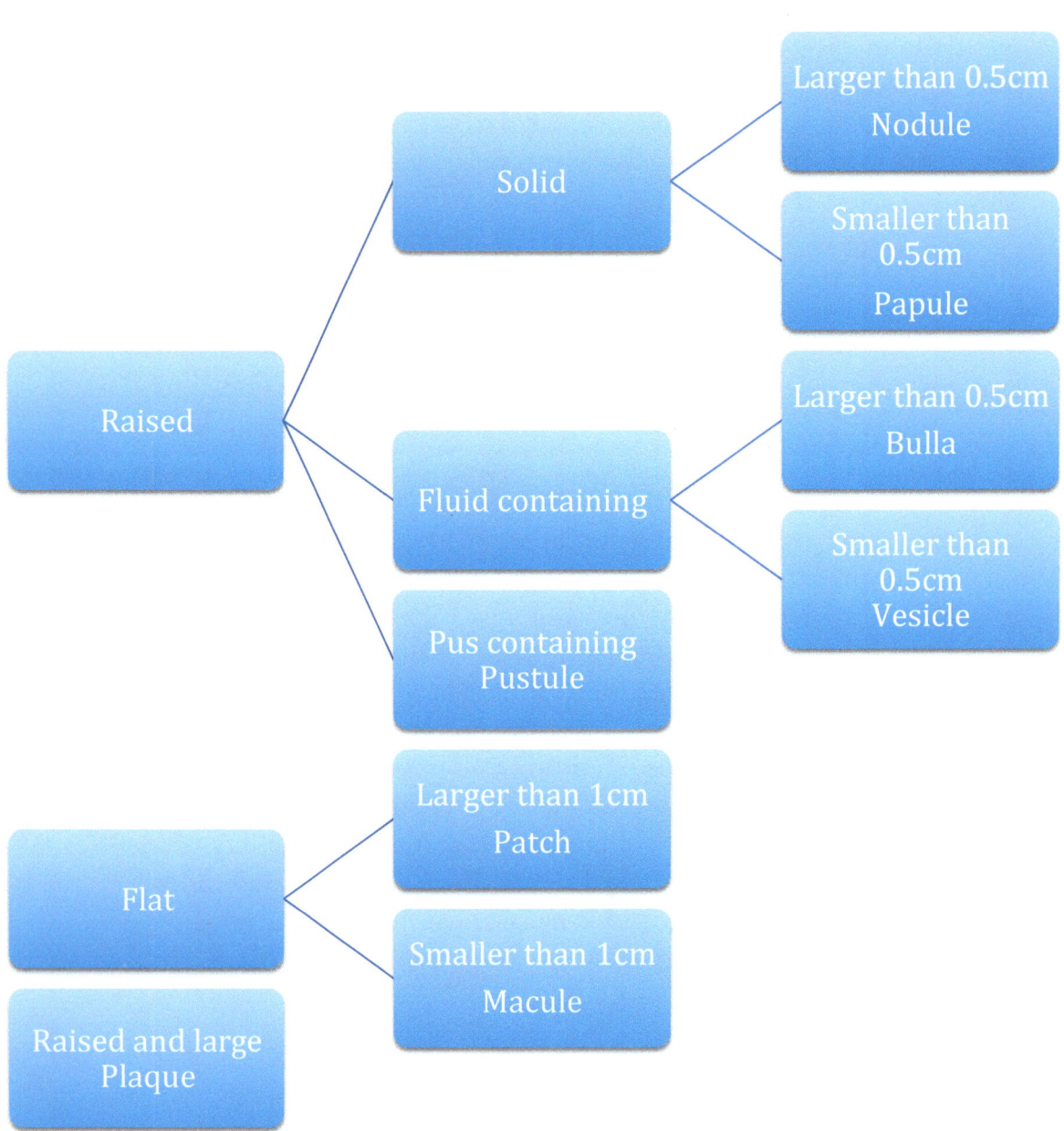

<u>Wheal:</u> Swelling in the upper epidermis of the skin

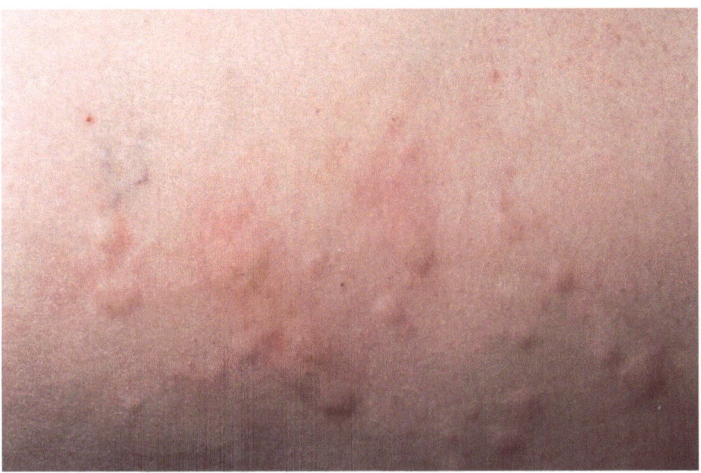

<u>Scale:</u> Visible flakes from epidermal shedding

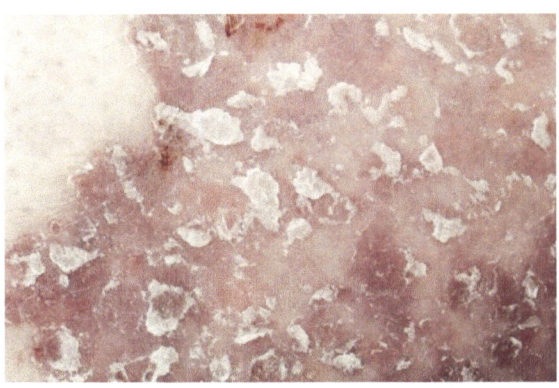

<u>Crust:</u> Dried exudate

<u>Horn:</u> A keratin projection

Burrow: Linear lesions/tunnels produced by a parasite like scabies.

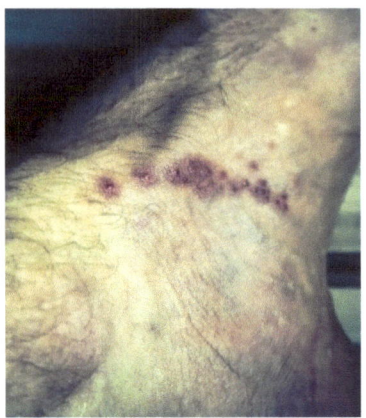

Lichenification: Thickening of the skin, usually from scratching.

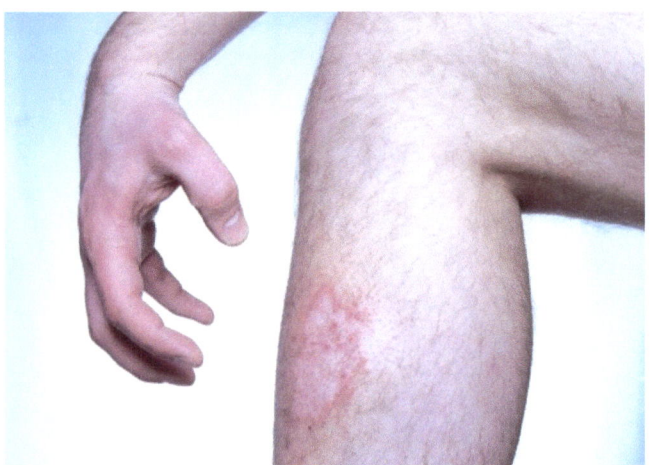

Telangiectasia: Dilatation of the skin's blood vessels, permanent.

Ecchymosis: Non-blanching bleeding in the skin.

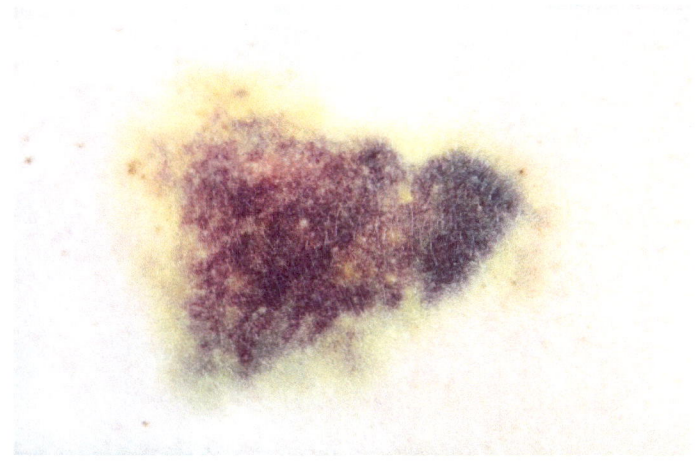

Petechiae: Small, 1-2mm bleed in the skin. Non-blanching

Purpura: Usually palpable lesions from bleeding in the skin. Non-blanching

Erosions: Loss of epidermis

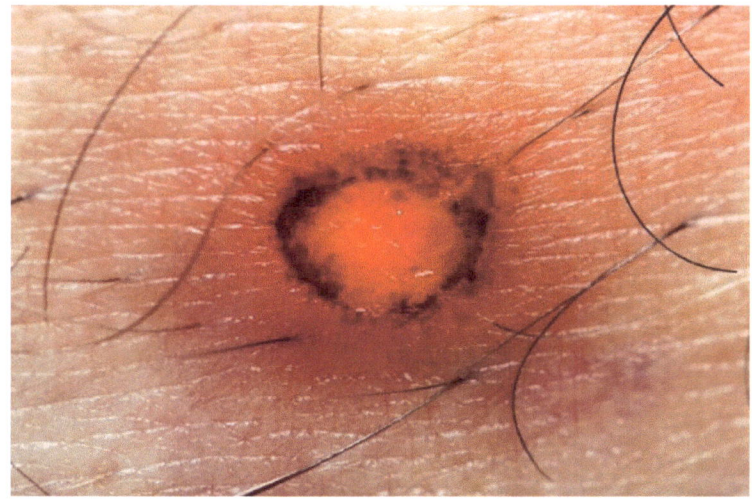

<u>Ulceration:</u> Loss of epidermis, dermis and sometimes subcutaneous tissue

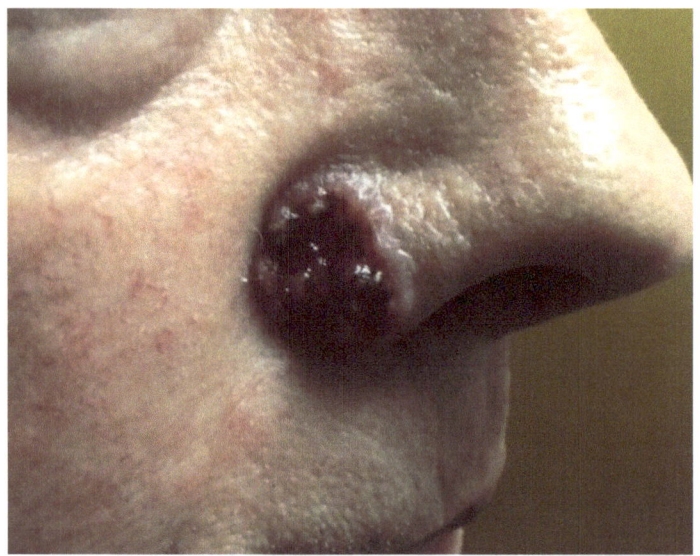

<u>Keloids:</u> Connective tissue formation that is more than necessary and extends beyond the border of the original wound.

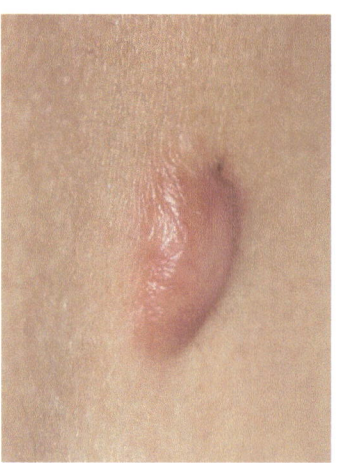

Pattern:

Discreet: Totally separate lesions

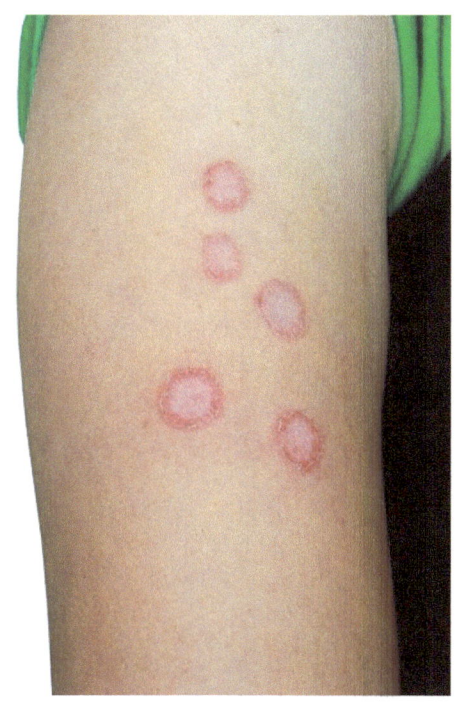

Clustered: Lesions that are grouped together

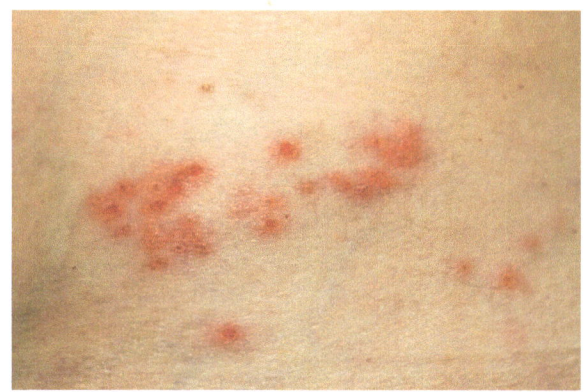

Annular: Lesions that are ring shaped/ circular

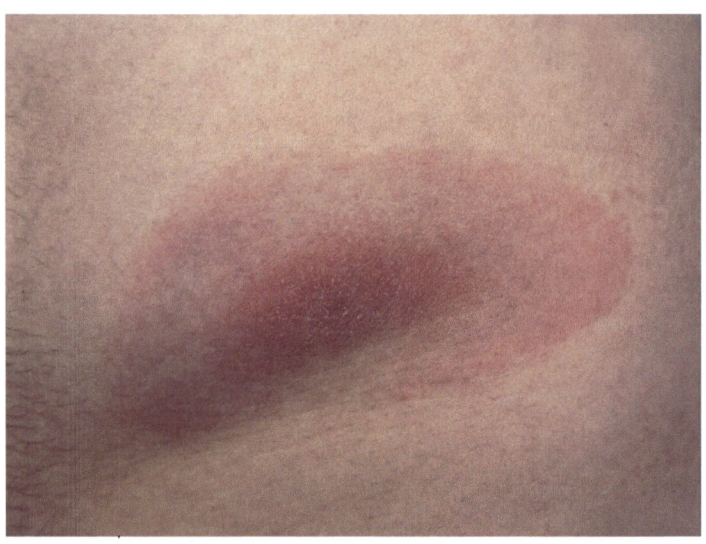

Dermatomal: Lesions following a dermatome distribution

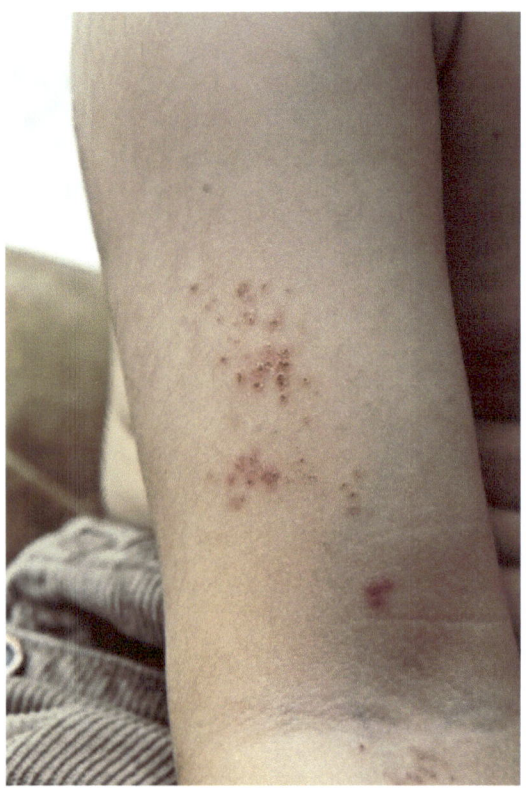

Guttate: Many small spots all over the skin.

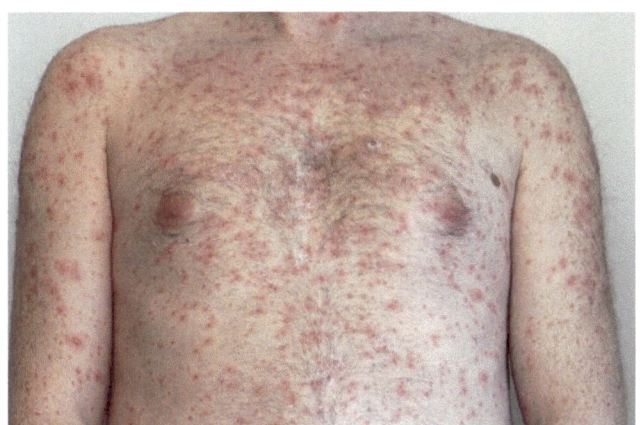

Anatomy of the skin

The human skin consists of 3 layers, the epidermis, dermis and subcutaneous tissue.

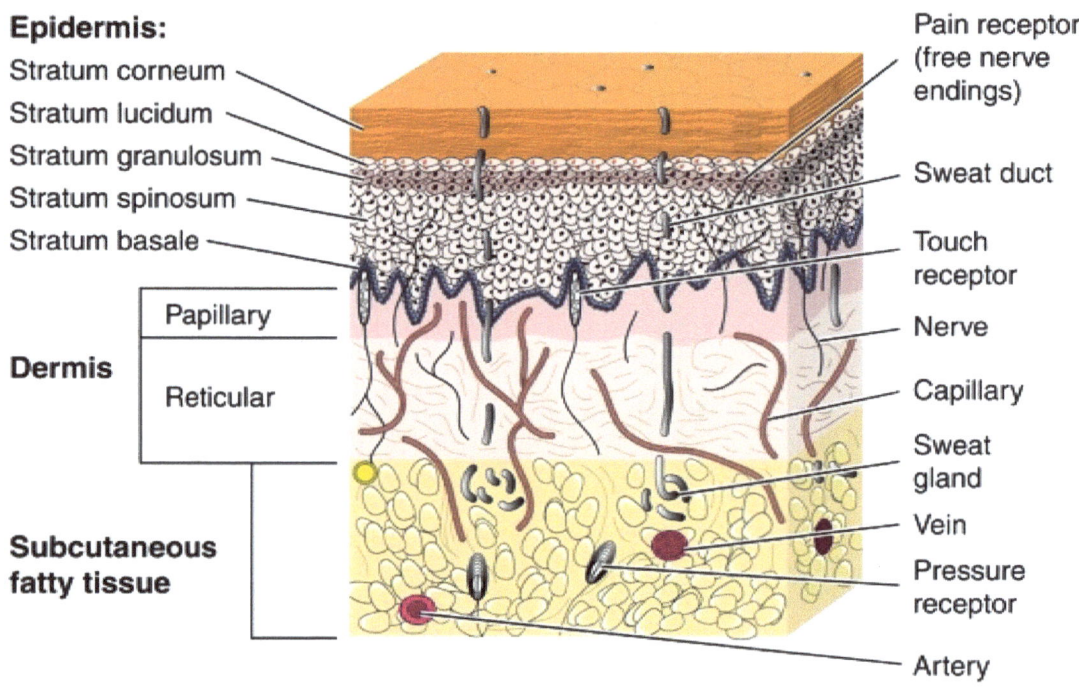

Epidermis:
Stratum corneum
Stratum lucidum
Stratum granulosum
Stratum spinosum
Stratum basale

Dermis
Papillary
Reticular

Subcutaneous fatty tissue

Pain receptor (free nerve endings)
Sweat duct
Touch receptor
Nerve
Capillary
Sweat gland
Vein
Pressure receptor
Artery

The epidermis is the outer layer of the skin and is stratified squamous epithelium. A single layer of basal cells forms the innermost part of the epidermis. Basal cells form keratinocytes that play an integral part in the body's defense system by creating an effective barrier. Keratinocytes migrate upwards to the surface of the skin and are gradually shed.
Melanocytes are scattered throughout the epidermis. They produce melanin, a pigment that gives skin its colour. Melanin filters UV rays and protects the skin from the sun. Langerhans cells in the epidermis form part of the body's immune system.

The dermis contains elastic (collagen, fibrillin and elastin fibers) and fibrous tissue. This level contains glands (sweat glands and sebaceous glands), hair follicles, nerve endings and blood vessels.

The deepest layer of the skin is the subcutaneous layer. It contains fat and connective tissues.

Acneiform eruptions and other pustules

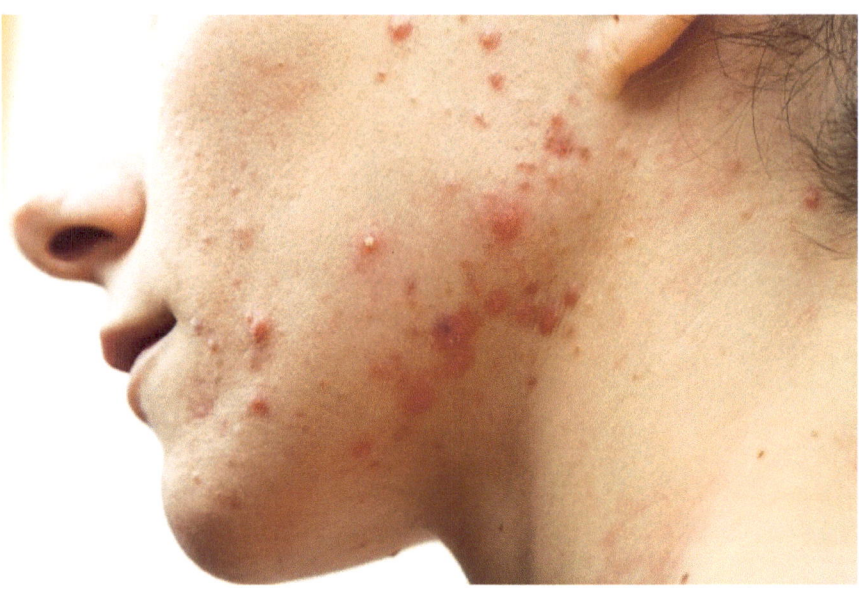

Acne vulgaris

Acne is frequently encountered in the primary care setting with patients stating the diagnosis without much uncertainty. It's a condition that plagued the human race since the beginning of mankind and is mentioned in Ancient Egyptian scripts. Even pharoahs struggled with this condition. Traces of an oil used to treat acne scars were found in King Tut's tomb.

Pathogenesis
Acne involves the pilosebaceous unit and is found where these units are present at highest concentrations i.e chin, cheeks, forehead, chest and the back. Sebaceous glands enlarge as a child reaches andrenarche, leading to an increase in the amount and severity of lesions

4 Steps are involved in the formation of acne:

1) Keratin plugs block the follicular canal.
2) Increased production of sebum in the pilosebaceous unit.
3) Proliferation of Proprionibacterium acnes (P.acnes), an anaerobe bacterium, which is part of the normal skin flora. Sebum is a growth medium for P. acnes.
4) Inflammation due to neutrophil action on the follicular wall. The wall becomes inflamed and weak. The contents end up moving into the dermis, causing an immune reaction, launched by the body towards the foreign matter that is now in the dermis of the skin. Pustules or cysts form due to this process.

Formation of Skin Pimples and Acne

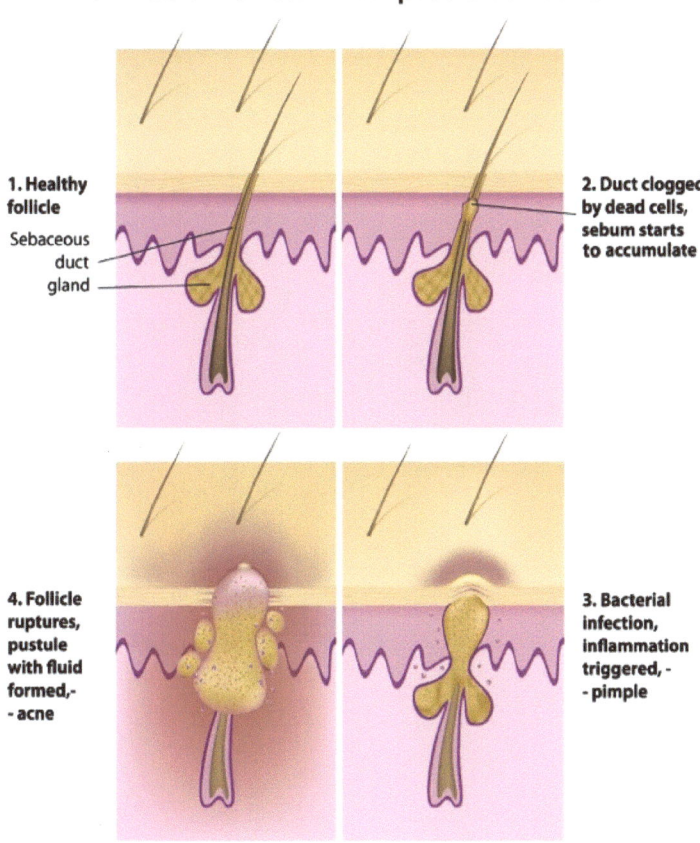

Clinical features

Acne is a clinical diagnosis. Patients have no problem identifying their condition and presents to you with the diagnosis already made. Acne can be classified into subgroups, depending on the severity and the clinical features.

Comedonal acne

This is most frequently encountered type of acne and consists of non-inflammatory lesions. P.acnes is not found in the overgrowth form. Comedonal acne can be either Open Comedones ("blackheads") or Closed Comedones ("whiteheads").

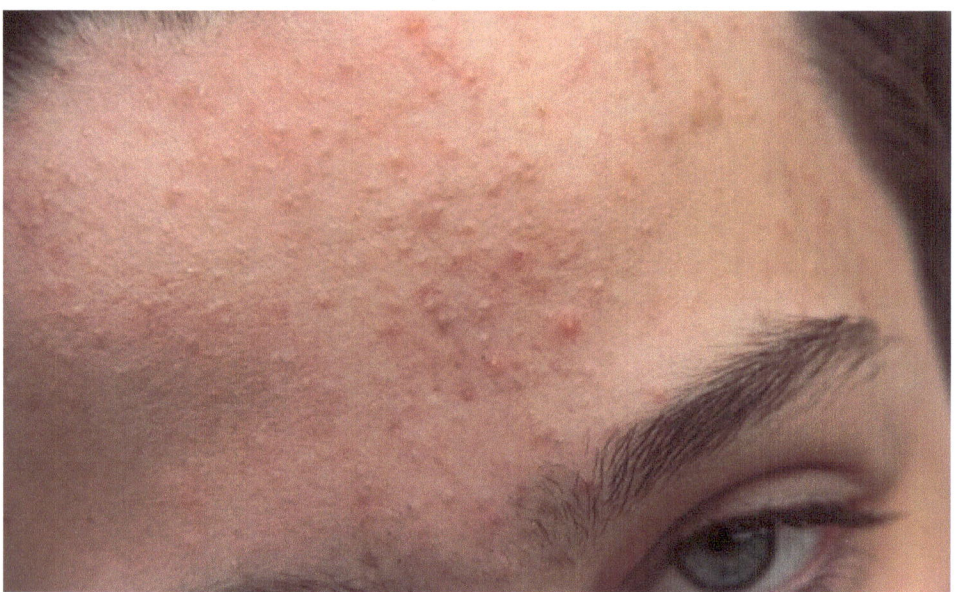

Closed comedones

Mild Inflammatory Acne

These lesions form when the comedones undergo an overgrowth of P.acnes. Fewer than 20 lesions on the body is classified as Mild Inflammatory Acne.

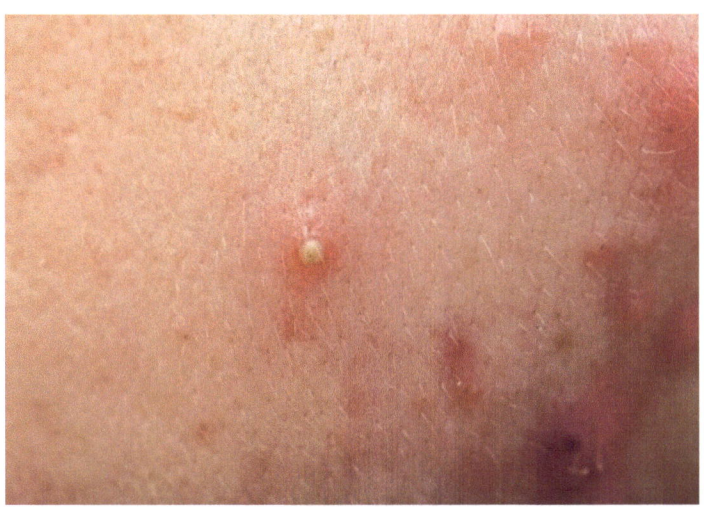

Mild inflammatory acne

Moderate To Severe Acne

This classification is reached when more than 20 pustules are present. This type of acne can lead to scarring.

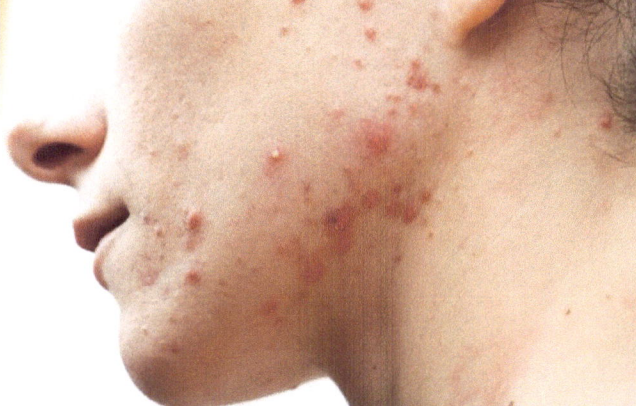

Moderate To Severe Acne

Nodulocystic acne

Nodulocystic acne is diagnosed when there is a large number of nodules and cysts present.

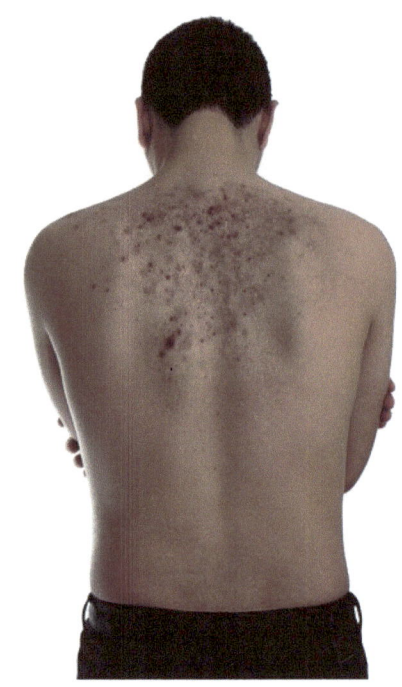

Nodulocystic acne

Treatment

Comedonal acne:
1) Topical retinoids
2) Topical azelaic acid
3) Topical salicylic acid

Mild Inflammatory acne:
1) Topical retinoids + Topical antimicrobial (e.g Clindamycin + tretinoin) + benzoyl peroxide
2) Oral antibiotics (Minocycline or Doxycycline) + topical retinoid
3) Alternative for females: Oral antiandrogens (Spironolactone)

Moderate to severe acne:
1) Oral antibiotics + Topical retinoids + benzoyl peroxide
2) Oral isotretinoin/ Alternative for females: Anti-androgens

Nodulocystic:
1) Oral isotretinoi
2) High dose oral antibiotics + topical retinoid

Retinoids:
1) Tretinoin – Retin A, Retin A Micro, Stieva
2) Isotretinoin – Accutane
3) Adapalene and Tazotrene

Benzoyl Peroxide combinations:
1) Benzoyl peroxide + erythromycin
2) Benzoyld peroxide + clindamycin
3) Benzoyl peroxide + dapsone

Oral antibiotics:
1) Minocycline: 50 to 100mg twice a day, tapered down after improvement of lesions.
2) Doxycycline: 100mg once to twice a day.
3) Clindamycin: 75mg to 300mg twice a day.
4) Tetracycline: 500mg twice a day until improvement, then 250mg twice a day.
5) Ampicillin or amoxicillin: 500mg twice a day.
6) Trimethoprim and Sulfamethoxazole: 160/800mg once or twice a day.

Anti-androgen therapy:
1) Oral contraceptives
2) Spironolactone: 50 to 200mg daily.

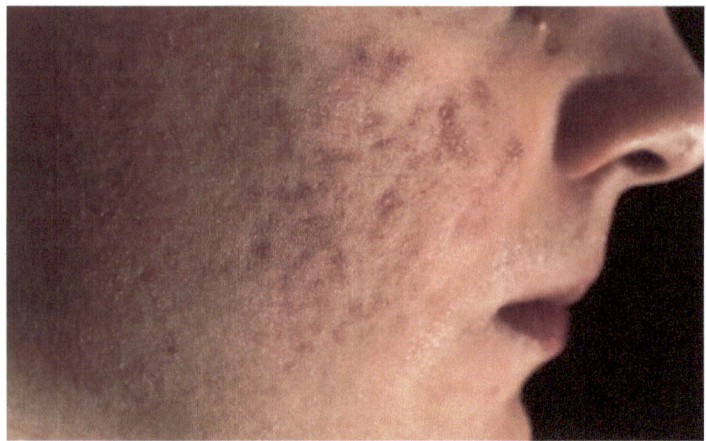

Acne scars

Pseudofolliculitis barbae

(ingrown hair)

Pseudofolliculitis barbae is a condition often seen in people who remove curly hair, especially with shaving. Papules and pustules form that can lead to scarring, pigment changes and superimposed bacterial infections.

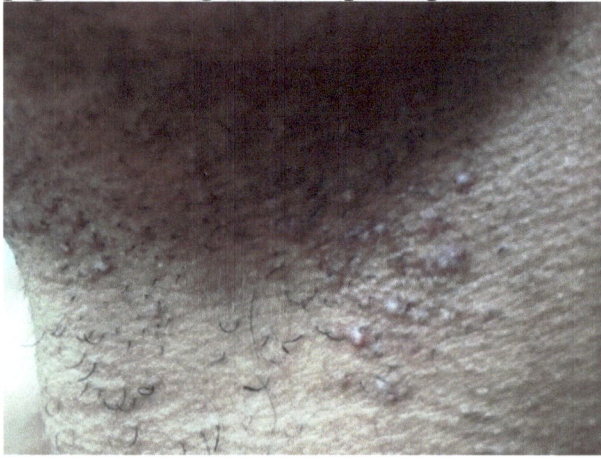

Treatment:
1) Discontinue shaving
2) Topical retinoids – tretinoin, adapalene (Differin gel®), tazarotene (Tazorac®)
3) Topical antimicrobials – Clindamycin, Erythromycin
4) Oral antibiotics in severe cases – Minocycline, Doxycycline and Tetracycline.

Hydradenitis supporitiva

This chronic disorder affects the folliculopilosebaceous units of the groin, axillae, perineum and perianal areas and can lead to abscesses, sinus tracts and scars. Genetics, obesity, smoking, hormones and certain drugs (levonorgestrel IUD) have been implicated in the pathogenesis of Hydradenitis supporitiva.

Clinical features
1) Open Comedones
2) Closed Comedones
3) Pustules
4) Scars
5) Sinus tracts

Treatment
Education about this chronic, recurring condition is the most important aspect of management.

Non-Pharmacological:
1) Smoke cessation
2) Weight reduction
3) Reduce high glycemic index foods and dairy
4) Hygiene

Pharmacological:
1) Topical antibiotics – clindamycin
2) Systemic antibiotics used for acne
   a) Doxycycline
   b) Minocycline
   c) Amoxacillin
   d) Clindamycin
3) Corticosteroid injections into the lesions
4) Anti-androgen therapy (Cyproterone acetate/Dianne)
5) Surgery, oral retinoids, TNF-alpha inhibitors.

Keratosis Pilaris

Abnormal follicular keratinization leads to a condition that is marked by perifollicular redness and small projections out of the follicle. This is called Keratosis Pilaris. The etiology is not fully known but genetics might play a role.

Clinical features
Keratosis Pilaris affects the extensor surfaces of the upper arms and thighs but it can spread to distal limbs and buttocks.

Treatment
1) Keratinolytics - lactic acid and salicylic acid
2) Emollients
3) Topical retinoids products – tretinoin, adapalene, tazotrene.

Perioral dermatitis

This condition falls in the group of acneiform disorders even though the term "dermatitis" is associated with eczematous rashes. Papules are found around the mouth, nose and sometimes the eyes. Topical steroids are often implicated in the pathogenesis of perioral dermatitis

Clinical features
1) Papules around the nasolabial fold and mouth with sparing of the skin of the lip adjacent to the vermillion border.
2) Burning sensation is often felt
3) No comedones are present
4) History of steroid use. Topical, inhaled or intranasal preparations

Treatment
1) Topical Calicneurin inhibitors – Pimecrolimus 1%
2) Metronidazole cream or gel
3) Erythromycin cream
4) Tetracycline 500mg twice a day until improvement and then 250 twice a day.
5) Oral Doxycycline 100mg once or twice a day.

6) Minocycline 50 to 100mg per day.

Treatment should be for 2 to 4 weeks and then tapered down over another 4 to 5 weeks.

Rosacea

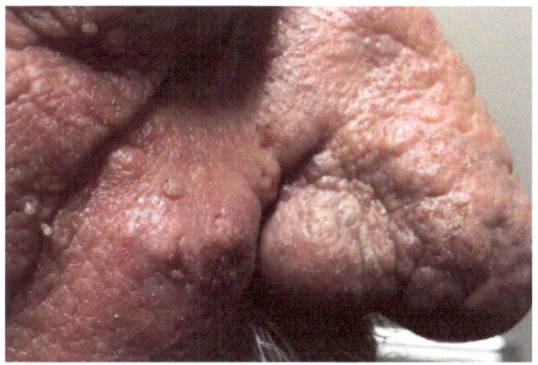

Rosacea patients complain that their face is too red and that they blush constantly. Rosacea is often worsened by spicy food, alcohol and emotional stress. Apart from the redness, they can also experience acne like pustules and nasal deformity. Ocular rosacea can occur in the absence of other manifestation and warrants referral to Ophthalmology. Symptoms include dry eyes, scratchy eyes, blepharitis and frequent conjunctivitis.

Clinical features of rosacea
1) Pustules – small monomorphic (all of the same size) papules and pustules.
2) Erythema
3) Sebaceous hyperplasia leading to enlargement of the nose (Rhinophyma)

Treatment
Non-Pharmacological:
Avoid triggers:
1) Sun exposure
2) Spicy foods
3) Alcohol
4) Extreme temperatures
5) Emotional stressors

Pharmacological:
1) Topical metronidazole
2) Topical azelaic acid
3) Topical clindamycin + benzoyl peroxide
4) Topical retinoids
5) Oral antibiotics (Doxycycline, Minocycline, Tetracycline)
6) Oral isotretinoin for patients failing to respond to above measures.

Miliaria (Heat rash)

Keratin plugs obstructing sweat glands at the stratum corneum level lead to build up of sweat in these units. This can lead to papules with erythema when the sweat leaks into the dermis (**Miliaria Rubra**). Miliaria can be papulopustular and non erythematous, known as miliaria profunda.

Miliaria pustulosa consists of more pustules with erythema.

Another form Miliaria that isn't pustular are **Miliaria crystalline** (vesicles without inflammation).

Treatment

Temperature control is the main form of treatment. The goal is to limit sweating. Other treatments that have documented benefits are topical steroids and topical antibiotics, menthol, calamine and lanolin.

Bacterial Infections

Impetigo

This contagious condition is most often seen in children. It is caused by staphylococcus aureus (bullous form) as well as streptococcus (non-bullous form). These lesions can start as a pustule but changes into the characteristic exudative crust. In the bullous form, large blisters develop with yellow fluid and cause exudation and crusting when they burst.

Differentiating these lesions from contact dermatitis is based on the symptoms: Impetigo is painful and dermatitis is itchy.

Treatment
Limited disease:
1) Topical mupirocin
2) Fusidic acid
3) Retapamulin
4) Hydrogen peroxide

Bullous lesions or extensive disease:
1) Dicloxacillin/ Cloxacillin 250-500 mg 6 hourly for 7 days
2) Clindamycin 15mg/kg/day 8 hourly for 10 days
3) Cephalexin 250mg every 6 hours for 7 days
4) Erythromycin 250-500 mg 6 hourly for 7 days
5) Azithromycin 500mg stat, then 250mg po daily for 4 days.

Cellulitis and erysipelas

Cellulitis is the infection of the subcutaneous tissues (deeper dermis and fat). The infected area becomes, red, swollen and hot. It can be with or without blisters. Onset is usually slower than erysipelas with fever following the erythema.

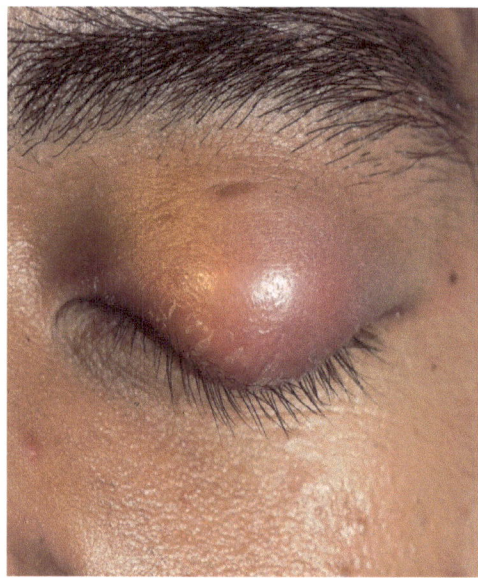

Cellulitis

Erysipelas is the infection of the upper dermis and superficial lymphatic system. Lesions are raised and well demarcated. Onset is more acute with fever and chills.

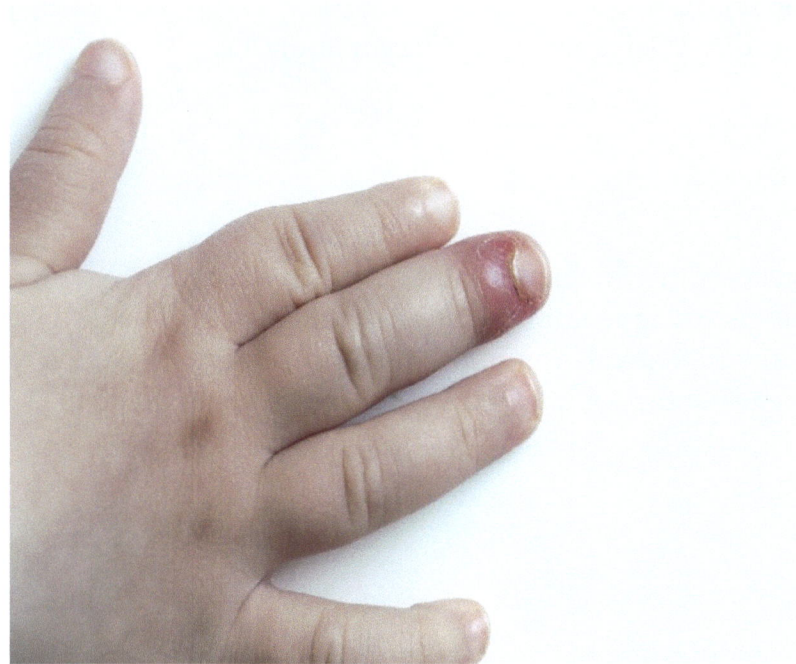

Erysipelas

Treatment

Elevate the limb to facilitate lymph drainage in both conditions.

Cellulitis:

Non-Purulent:

1) Cephalexin 500mg 6 hourly for 5 days
2) Clindamycin 300mg 6 to 8 hourly for 5 to 10 days
3) Amoxacillin 500 8 hourly + TMP/SMX (800/160mg 1 to 2 twice a day for 5 to 10 days)
4) Amoxacillin 500mg 8 hourly + Doxycycline/ Minocycline for 5 to 10 days

Purulent:

1) Clindamycin 300mg 6 to 8 hourly for 5 to 10 days.
2) TMP/SMX 800/160MG 1 to 2 twice a day for 5 to 10 days
3) Doxycycline 100mg twice a day for 5 to 10 days
4) Minocycline 100mg twice a day for 5 to 10 days

Erysipelas:
1) Amoxacillin 500mg 8hourly
2) Penicillin 500mg 6 hourly
3) Erythromycin 250mg 6 hourly
4) Ceftriaxone 1g IV per day/ Cefazolin 1-2g every 8 hours IV

Erythrasma

Erythrasma is an infection caused by the bacterium Corynebacterium minutissimum (Gram positive) and is seen in the intertriginous areas. The condition can occur in healthy individuals but immunocompromised, the elderly, diabetic patients, obese patients and people living in the tropics are at greater risk.

Clinical features
1) Well defined patch
2) Erythematous to brown
3) Sometimes plaque-like appearance
4) Scaling and wrinkling of the skin.

Diagnosis can be confirmed with a Wood's lamp with a coral-red/pink fluorescence.

Treatment
Topical:
1) Clindamycin +- Benzoyl Peroxide
2) Fusidic acid
3) Miconazole, Tioconazole

Oral treatment: For widespread disease: Clarithromycin, Erythromycin

Ecthyma

This is an infection caused by staphylococcus aureus or streptococcus. It is more common in patients who are immunocompromised, diabetics, alcoholics and intravenous drug abusers.

Clinical features
Annular, ulcerative lesions that are well demarcated

Treatment
1) Penicillin V 500mg 6 hourly for 2 weeks
2) Flucloxacillin 500mg 6 hourly for 2 weeks

Pitted keratolysis

This is an infection of the horny layer in the skin of the feet. This condition, which is often wrongly diagnosed as warts, is associated with excess moisture and sweating of the feet.

Treatment
Topical antibiotics:
1) Clindamycin
2) Fusidic acid

Bacterial folliculitis, carbuncles and furuncles

Staphylococcus aureus is often implicated in the formation of pustules with an erythematous base, a condition called folliculitis.
 When there is a coalescence of these infected follicles, a carbuncle forms. Folliculitis and carbuncles only involve the epidermis. The dermis is spared. If the infection spreads to the dermis, a furuncle (boil) forms.

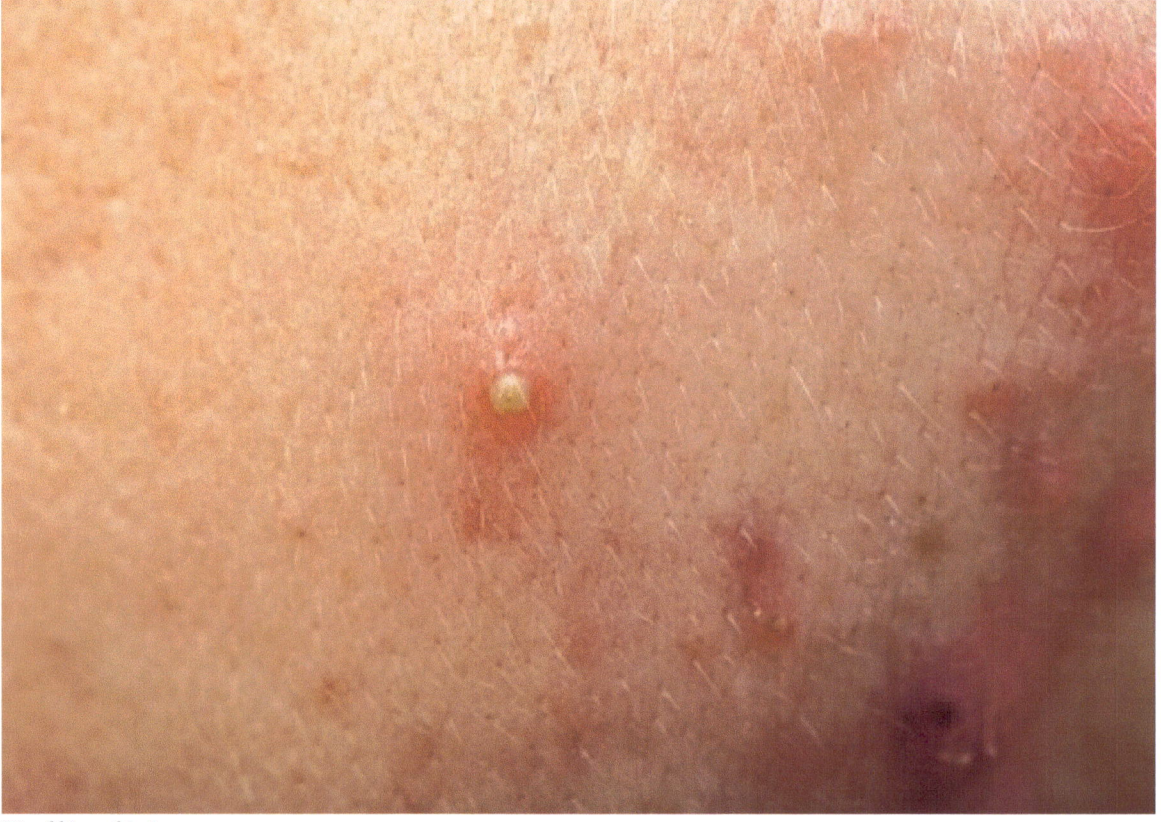

Folliculitis

Treatment

Folliculitis:
Mupirocin ointment

Carbuncles and Furuncles:
Drainage
If antibiotics are considered, it should be effective against MRSA based on culture and sensitivity results.
Choices are:
1) TMP/SMX 160/800 to 320/1600 mg twice a day
2) Minocycline 100mg twice a day
3) Doxyxycline 100mg twice a day
4) Clindamycin 300mg 6 to 8 hourly

Fungal Infections

Fungal infections can be subdivided into molds (tinea infections) and yeasts (candida and seborrheic dermatitis)

Tinea (Dermatophyte) infections

Three types of dermatophytes cause the majority of tinea infections.
These dermatophytes are:
1) *Epidermophyton*
2) *Trichophyton*
3) *Microsporum*

Tinea infections are named according to the area of the body that is affected:
Tinea pedis – affecting the feet
Contact with infected keratin debris in showers and pools are the main causes for the spread of this form of tinea.

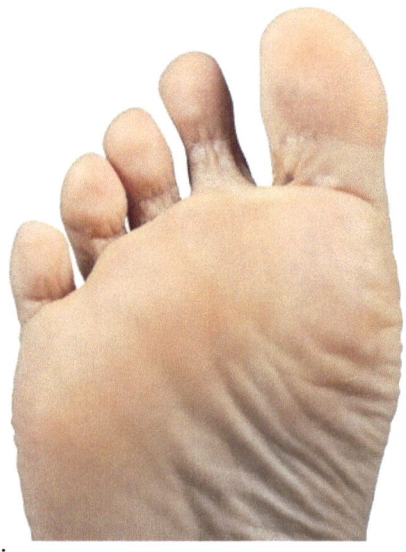

Tinea pedis

Tinea capitis – scalp infection.

This is more common in children due to the fungistatic nature of fatty acids in post pubertal sebum.

Tinea cruris – groin infection.
Often transferred from the feet by scratching fingers or towels.

Tinea corporis - arms and legs affected.
Tinea can affect any part of the body even though it's seen less often.

Tinea unguium – nail infection.
Toenails are more commonly affected than fingernails and the big toe nails more often than the other toes.

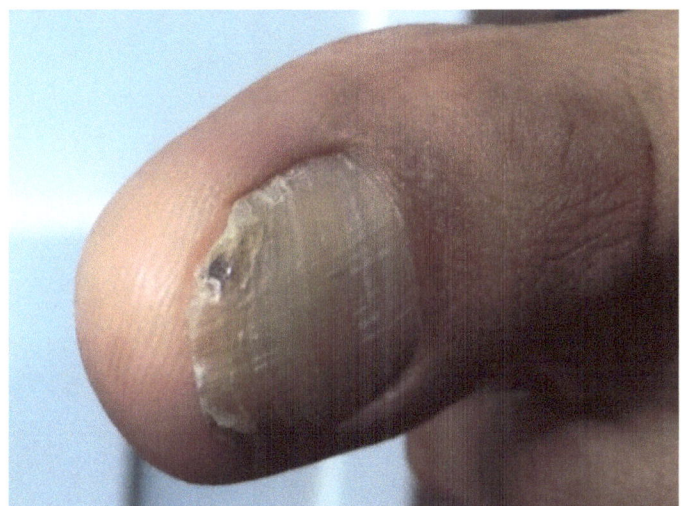

Tinea unguium

Tinea manuum – hand affected

Clinical features
1) Well defined and demarcated lesion
2) Erythematous
3) Looks psoriasiform on the limbs
4) Often with central clearing

Diagnosis
Hair, nail clippings and skin scrapings can be tested by KOH examination and culture
Wood's lamp: Hairs show silver-blue/green fluorescence.

Treatment

<u>Tinea Pedis, Tinea cruris, Tinea corporis and tinea manuum</u>
1) Terbinafine 1% cream twice a day for 1 week
2) Butenafine cream twice a day for 1 weeks
3) Ciclopirox cream twice a day for up to 4 weeks
4) Ketoconazole cream twice a day for 6 weeks

<u>Extensive disease:</u>
1) Terbinafine 250mg daily for 2 weeks
2) Itraconazole 200mg twice daily for one week
3) Fluconazole 150mg weekly for 6 weeks
4) Griseovulfin 1000mg per day for up to 6 weeks (less effective than other oral antifungals)

<u>Tinea capitis:</u>
1) Griseofulvin 500mg daily orally for 4 to 6 weeks is as effective as Terbinafine with a slight advantage over certain tinea species.
2) Terbinafine 250mg once a day for 6 weeks
3) Fluconazole 150mg weekly for 6 weeks.

<u>Tinea unguium:</u>
Oral treatment is recommended:
1) Terbinafine 250mg daily for 6 weeks (fingernails) and 12 weeks (toenails)
2) Itraconazole 200mg daily for 12 weeks for toenails and 200mg daily for 1 week for fingernails, with a repeat course after a 3 week drug free period.

Tinea barbae

Fungal infections of the beard can lead to pustules with typical tinea like annular configurations.

Treatment

Oral antifungals e.g terbinafine, griseofulvin or itraconazole should be used.
1) Terbinafine 250mg/day for 2 to 4 weeks
2) Griseofulvin 500mg daily for 2-6 weeks
3) Itraconazole 100mg daily for 14 days or 200mg daily for 7 days

Candida

Candida albicans is responsible for the most yeast infections and affects the skin and mucous membranes.
Risk factors for candida infections include immunosuppression (lymphoma, chemotherapy, HIV/AIDS, corticosteroid treatment), diabetes, pregnancy, topical steroid creams, antibiotic therapy, and apposition of the skin to produce a suitable environment.
The most common infections are:
Vulvovaginal candida and **Balanitis.**

Pruritic, white discharge leads to painful and swollen vaginal. In men, Candida will present as white patches and erosions in the mucosa, more often in uncircumcised men. Testing the urine for glucose is advised in anyone with signs of vulvovaginitis or balanitis.

Treatment
Topical: Miconazole 2% cream
Vaginal treatment: a) Miconazole 1 to 3 days
                   b) Nystatin daily for 7 days
                   c) Clotrimazole 3 to 7 days
Oral therapies: Fluconazole 150mg single dose

Oral candida

Oral candida is part of normal oral flora in many adults but candidiasis is often associated with immunosuppression, diabetes, broad-spectrum antibiotics, inhaled corticosteroids, and certain cancers. Oropharyngeal candidiasis is seen in HIV patients and extremely common in people with AIDS.
White plaques form on the mucosa of the mouth. The oral mucosa becomes inflamed and sore. Scraping these plaques will show inflamed epithelium underneath that will bleed easily.

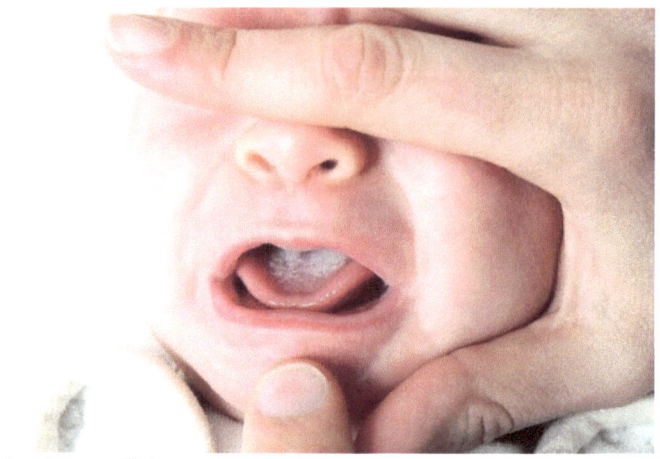
Oral candida

Treatment
1) Nystatin pastilles 1 to 2 orally 4 to 5 times a day for 1 week or as needed
2) Fluconazole 200mg daily orally for 7 days
3) Ketoconazole 200mg per day for 2 weeks
4) Itraconazole 100 to 200mg daily for 3 to 4 weeks.

Intertrigo

Intertrigo develops when two apposing skin surfaces create a moist and warm environment for candida species to flourish. The areas most commonly affected are:
1) Under the breast
2) Axillae
3) Underneath the abdominal fat apron in obese patients
4) Groins
5) Intergluteal folds
6) Neck folds in infants

Clinical features
1) Erythematous patches or plaques
2) Macerated appearance
3) Satellite lesions, tiny pustules at the border of the lesion

Treatment

Topical treatment:
1) Ketoconazole
2) Miconazole
3) Clotrimazole
4) Tebinafine
5) Ciclopirox

Drying agents: Powders containing tolnaftate, nystatin and miconazole

Oral therapy:
1) Fluconazole 150mg weekly
2) Itraconazole 200mg twice daily

Candida nail infections (paronychia)

Candida nail infections are more common in people whose occupations require them to have their hand immersed in water for extended periods. The proximal nail fold and matrix becomes infected, leading to inflammation and distortion of the nail.

Clinical features
1) Loss of cuticle
2) Thickening of the nail
3) Discoloration of the nail
4) Nail dystrophy
5) Erythema of the proximal nail fold

Treatments

Corticosteroid and imidazole cream combinations - ketoconazole 2% in betamethasone 0.05% twice a day for duration of condition.

Seborrheic dermatitis

Little is known about the pathogenesis of seborrheic dermatitis but Malassezia yeast is often implicated in the formation of this common rash. The rash follows the pattern of the sebaceous gland distribution in the skin and is most often seen on the forehead, nasolabial folds, eyebrows and glabella, eyelids, axillae and scalps of babies. The effect of maternal androgens on sebum glands on the scalps of babies is considered as the cause for seborrheic dermatitis of the scalp or "cradle cap".

Clincial features
1) Scaling
2) Erythematous patches and plaques
3) Sometimes mild pruritus
4) Distinctive distribution of the "T" of the face, scalp of babies, axillae and eyelids.

Treatment
Cradle cap (babies):
1) Hydrocortisome 1% cream once a day for a week
2) Ketoconazole 2% cream or shampoo twice a week for 2 weeks

Face and trunk seborrheic dermatitis:
1) Ketoconazole 2% cream or gel twice a day for 4 weeks
2) Ciclopirox 1% gel twice a day for 4 weeks

Scalp (Adults):
1) Ketoconazole 2% shampoo twice a week for 8 weeks
2) Ciclopirox 1% shampoo twice a week for 4 weeks

Tinea versicolor

(Pityriasis versicolor)

Tinea versicolor is an infection caused by the fungus Malassezia globosa (most common) and Malassezia furfur, lipid-dependent yeasts. Malassezia fungus is part of the normal flora of the skin and is not associated with poor hygiene. It is not considered contagious but rather is a result with excessive sweating and more often seen during warmer weather.

Clinical features

1) Well demarcated macules with slight scale
2) Hypopigmented lesions due to melanocyte damage.
3) Hyperpigmented lesions (in lighter skins usually)
4) Erythematous macules
5) Trunk and upper limbs mostly affected

Diagnosis

Obtaining skin scrapings and examine it with potassium hydroxide will show a "spaghetti-and-meatballs" pattern.
Wood's lamp will reveal yellow-white to yellow-green fluorescence.

Treatment

Topical:
1) Ketoconazole 2% cream once daily for 14 days
2) Ketoconazole 2% shampoo, lather for 5 minutes and then rinse daily for 2 weeks
3) Terbinafine cream twice a day for 2 weeks
4) Ciclopirox 1% cream twice a day for 4 weeks.
5) Selenium 2.5% lotion applied for 10 minutes per day for 7 days.

Selenium 1% shampoo is often recommended but seems to be less effective than the 2.5% lotion.

Systemic therapy
1) Itraconazole 200mg orally per day for 7 days
2) Fluconazole 300mg once a week for 2 weeks/ 150mg per week for 4 weeks
3) Ketoconazole 200mg daily for 5 days

Eczematous and erythematous lesions

Eczema

Eczema is probably the most common disorder you'll encounter in your practice. It can be classified into:
1) Atopic dermatitis
2) Irritant contact dermatitis
3) Allergic contact dermatitis
4) Lichen simplex chronicus
5) Nummular eczema

Atopic Dermatitis:

This chronic inflammatory disorder is part of the atopic triad of eczema, asthma and allergic rhinitis. Genetics is involved in the formation of these lesions. Approximately 5 to 20% of children are affected throughout the world and the incidence seems to be on the incline. The pathogenesis is largely based on an impairment of the epidermal barrier and an inflammatory response due to outside factors.

Triggering factors include:
1) Change in temperature and humidity
2) Excessive washing
3) Irritant substances
4) Food – milk, fish, eggs, wheat, peanuts
5) Emotional stress

Clinical features
1) Erythema
2) Pruritus and excoriations
3) Scaly skin
4) Erosions
5) Exudations

6) Papules
7) More common in flexural areas

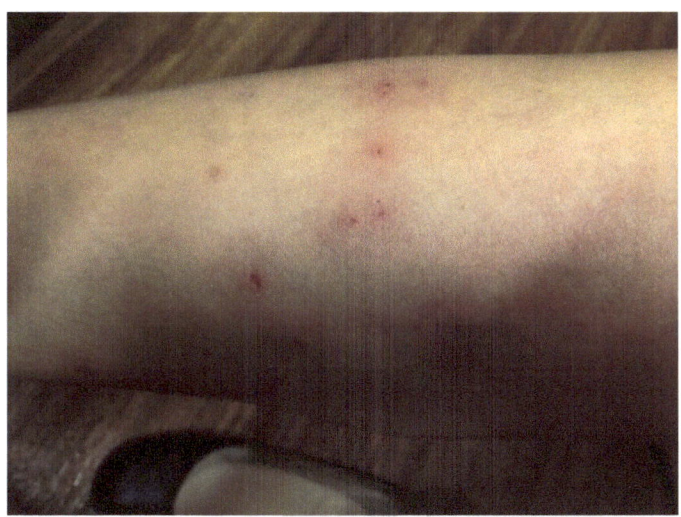

Atopic dermatitis with excoriations

Common Sites of Eczema in Children and Adults

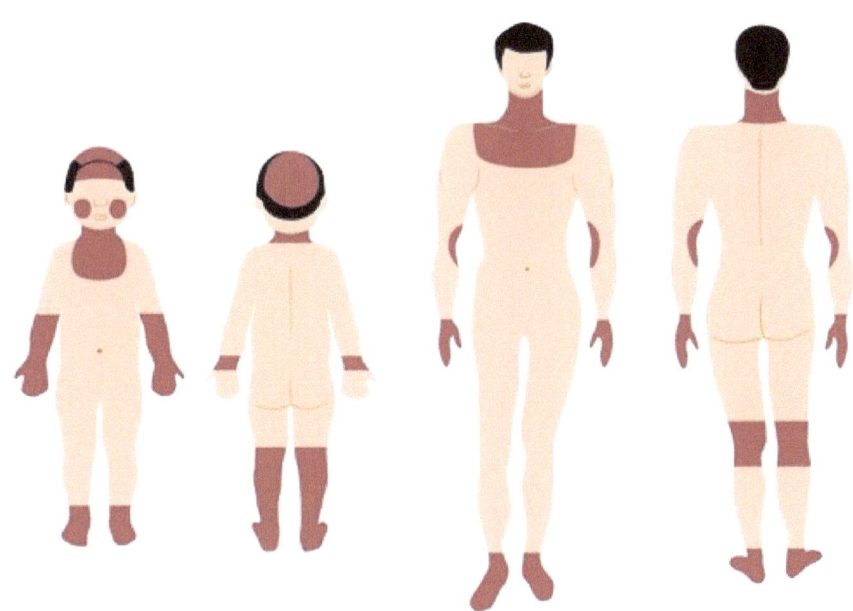

Treatment

1) Avoid triggers
2) Treat pruritus with sedative antihistamines (Hydroxyzine, diphenhydramine)
3) Moisturize skin (Nutraderm, Eucerin, Cetaphil, petroleum jelly, Vaseline)

4) Topical corticosteroids
5) Topical calcineurin inhibitors
6) Severe cases can be treated with oral prednisone, cyclosporine, combined UVA/UVB, Psoralen UVA, Narrowband UVB light therapy and triamcinolone.
7) Oral antibiotics should be used for superimposed infections. Treatment is targeted to Staphylococcus aureus.
    a. Cephalexin 250mg 6 hourly
    b. Flucloxacillin 500mg 6 hourly

Choice of topical steroids
Mild disease:
Low potency steroid - hydrocortisone 2.5%
Moderate disease:
Moderate potency steroids - Triamcinolone 0.1%, betamethasone dipropionate 0.05%
Severe disease:
High/ Super high potency steroids - clobetasol proprionate

Treatment is for 2 weeks and a lower potency steroid or calcineurin inhibitor should be used for maintenance treatment.
Topical calcineurin inhibitors:
Pimecrolimus or Tacrolimus (0.1% or 0.03%).
These agents are considered to be equally in strength to medium potency steroids.

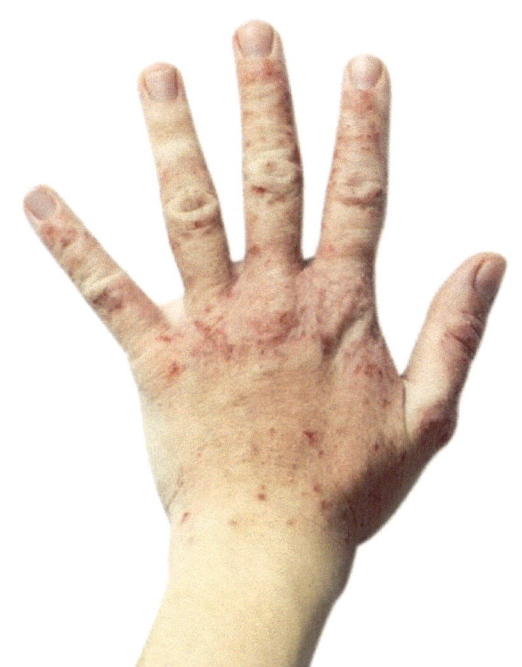

Severe hand eczema

Irritant contact dermatitis

Contact irritant dermatitis is caused or aggravated by repeated hand washing or patients in contact with chemicals. It is commonly found in nurses, doctors, dishwashers, cleaners and fishermen. Irritants like water, detergents, solvents, acids and alkalis disrupt the protective function of the stratum corneum that leads to increased water loss.

Clinical features:
1) Dry skin
2) Cracked skin
3) Erythema
4) Swelling of the hands
5) Pain and even bleeding
6) Pruritus
7) Vesicles

Treatment:
1) Avoidance of irritant by wearing gloves, gentle washing,
2) Moisturize: Petrolium, Lanolin, ceramides.
3) Topical corticosteroids:
   a) Mild disease: High Potency - betamethasone diproprionate twice a day for two to 4 weeks.
   b) Severe disease: Super High Potency e.g Clobetasol proprionate twice a day for 2 to 4 weeks.

Allergic contact dermatitis

This disorder is a T cell-mediated allergic response or a type VI delayed hyperactivity reaction. The most common causes are:
   a) Nickel
   b) Chromium
   c) Gold
   d) Cobalt
   e) Formaldehyde
   f) Balsam of Peru
   g) Topical antibiotics
   h) Topical steroids
   i) Rubber
   j) Sodium Thiosulfate
   k) Hair dyes

Clinical features
   1) Erythema
   2) Plaques
   3) Vesicles
   4) Edema
   5) Lesions location corresponds with area exposed to allergen

Patch testing should be used to determine the exact allergen responsible for the rash.

Treatment
   1) Avoid exposure to allergen
   2) Topical corticosteroids
   3) Topical calcineurin inhibitors (Pimecrolimus, Tacrolimus)
   4) Systemic corticosteroids when large body surface area affected
   5) Oral antihistamines

Nummular eczema

Nummular eczema lesions are round, erythematous plaques and may resemble psoriasis. The cause is not clear but the treatment is the same as for atopic dermatitis.

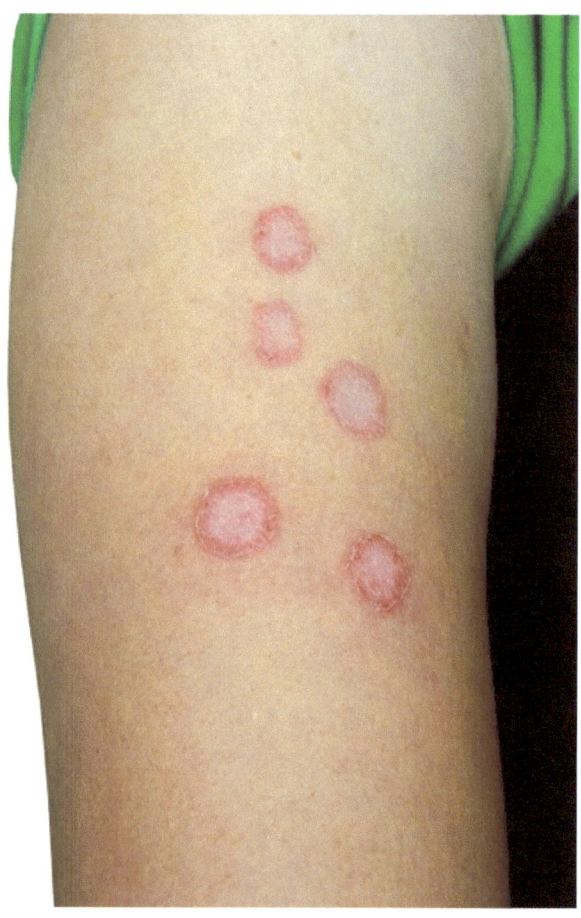

Lichen simplex chronicus (Neurodermatitis)

Lichen simplex chronicus plaques form due to a chronic itch-scratch cycle. An unknown irritant can start the scratching that leads to the lichenification of the skin. The most common sites are wrists, shins, back of the neck and palms.

Treatment
Treatment is aimed at breaking the itch-scratch cycle, sometimes by means of occlusion and potent topical steroids but treatment is often unsatisfactory.

Other erythematous lesions

Pityriasis rosea

This common, self-limiting condition of unclear etiology causes a distinctive pattern of papulosquamous lesions. It affects the trunk and proximal limbs with oval erythematous patches. Human Herpes viruses 6,7 and 8 have all been implicated in the pathogenesis but without overwhelming evidence.

Clinical features
1) A mild prodromal illness precedes the rash
2) A single, round, well demarcated, pink "Herald" patch of 2 to 5 cm appears on the back, neck or chest
3) The "Herald" patch begins to resolve and leads to an eruption of crops of smaller patches less than 2 weeks later.
4) Distributions include the trunk and proximal upper and lower limbs.
5) The long axis of the lesions lie in lines running from the back to the front (Langer's lines) leading to the "Christmas tree" distribution.
6) Scale of each lesion tends to peel from the inside towards the border
7) Lesions resolve in 6 to 8 weeks.

Treatment
This condition is self-limiting and no treatment is needed.
Pruritus can be controlled with topical corticosteroids (Betamethasone diproprionate 0.05%, Hydrocortisone 1%)
Erythromycin 250mg 4 times a day has been tried with little evidence of effect.
Acyclovir 800mg five times a day for 7 days can shorten the duration of the lesions.

Granuloma annulare

Erythematous plaques usually form on the trunk and distal extremities of patients with granuloma annulare. This is a self-limiting condition with unknown etiology and can last for months to years. Insect bites, viral infections, sun exposure and drugs have all been implicated in the pathogenesis of this condition but the evidence is lacking.

Clinical features of lesions
1) Erythematous plaques
2) Annular shape
3) Central clearing
4) Asymptomatic
5) Palms, soles, head and neck are usually spared
6) Trunk and extremities are usually affected

Associated disorders
Diabetes, malignancies (lymphoma), thyroids disease, HIV and lipid disorders have all been associated with a granuloma annulare rash.

Treatment
1) Topical corticosteroids (high potency e.g clobetasol) once to twice a day for 4 weeks.
2) Intralesional corticosteroids (triamcinolone)
3) Topical calcineurin inhibitors (Tacrolimus 0.1% or ppimecrolimus) twice a day for 4 to 6 weeks.
4) Phototherapy, isotretinoin, hydroxychloroquine and dapsone can be initiated at specialist level.

Erythema multiforme

This common condition is often a result of viruses (Herpes simplex being the most common virus), radiotherapy, other infections (bacterial and fungal), or medication. It is a process of vasculitis.

Clinical features

1) May be associated with a prodromal phase of fever and malaise
2) "Target" or "iris" lesions form characterized by:
    a. Round or oval shapes
    b. Maculopapular appearance
    c. Lesions have a purplish center.
    d. Centre can become vesicular or cyanotic.
    e. Extensor aspects of the arms, legs, hands and feet are most widely affected
3) Lesions heal within 3 weeks

Treatment

It is a self-limiting condition and mild cases are not treated.

More widespread lesions can be treated with a course of prednisone for 2 weeks.

Trial of Acyclovir 400mg twice a day for 1 to 2 weeks can be effective.

Insect bites

Bed Bugs

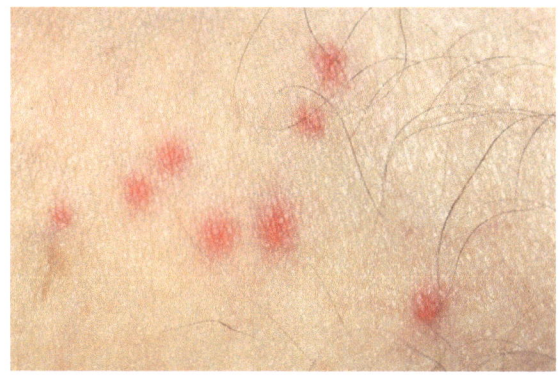

These insects emerge just before dawn and bites the exposed areas of the skin. The reaction of the bite causes a 2-5mm papular rash with urticaria (wheals) and can even lead to blistering. It can take 0 to 10 days for the rash to appear and will resolve in 7 days if untreated. Getting rid of the insects can be obtained by fumigation of the house.

Treatment

Treatment isn't necessary but in cases where the lesions cause severe discomfort, topical corticosteroid creams and antihistamines (systemic) will be beneficial.

Head lice (Pediculosis capitis)

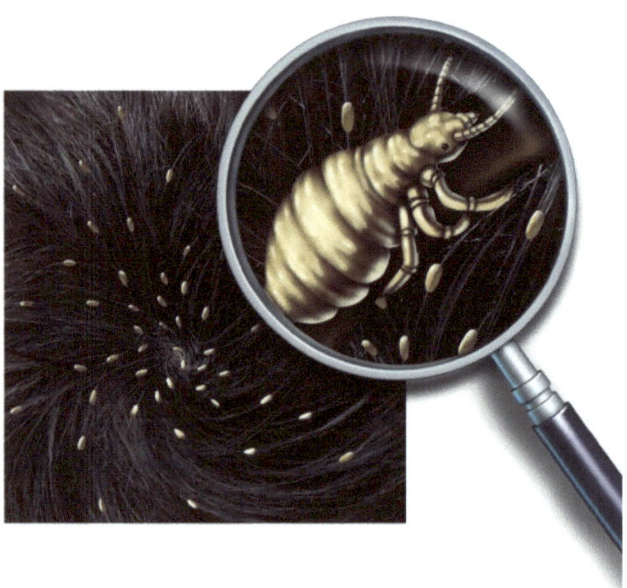

This wingless insect spreads when there is head-to-head contact with an infected individual.

Clinical features
1) Itching
2) Nits (eggs)

Treatment
1) Permethrin 1% applied to washed hair. Leave on and rinse after 10minutes. Repeat after 1 week if necessary.
2) Malanthion applied to hair and left on for 12 hours. Repeat after one week if necessary
3) Lindaine applied to hair and left for 4 minutes to lather
4) Spinosad applied to dry hair. Repeat if necessary after 7 days

Urticaria

Urticaria is the formation of hives often due to the release of histamine from mast cells. The lesions are pruritic and erythematous and can be associated with angioedema. Angioedema is due to submucosal or subcutaneous swelling. Urticaria is subdivided as acute urticarial, chronic urticarial, physical urticarias, hereditary angioedema, and urticarial pigmentosa. The lesions always resolve within 24 hours. When lesions last more than 24 hours, a vasculitic cause should be considered.

Clinical picture
1) Well circumscribed
2) Raised erythematous lesions
3) Can have central pallor
4) Very itchy

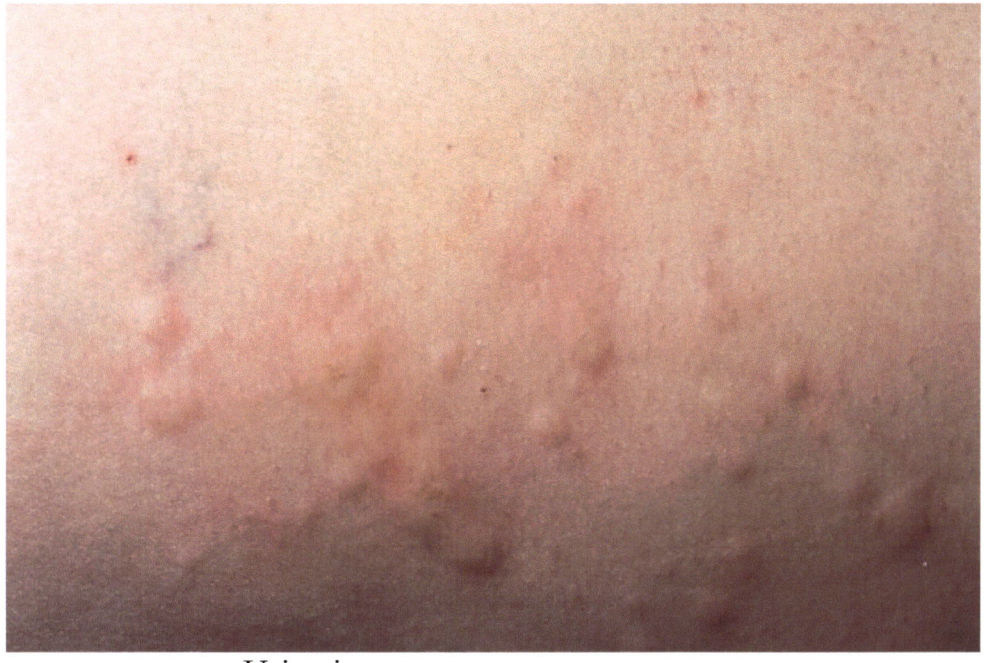
Uricaria

Acute urticaria

If the condition resolves within 6 weeks, it's considered acute urticarial. It is usually caused by an allergic reaction to plants, insect bites, medications (aspirin, penicillin) and foods, or due to viral and bacterial infections.

Treatment
1) Non-sedating H1 antihistamines as first line. Certirizine 10mg daily
2) Sedating/ First generation H1 antihistamine. Hydroxyzine 25 to 50 mg daily. Diphenhydramine 25 to 50 mg daily or as needed
3) Oral prednisone 30 to 60mg, tapering own over 1 week.

Chronic urticaria

Chronic idiopathic urticarial is a condition characterized by urticarial lesions on most days of the week for six weeks or longer. In most cases there is no known external allergic cause. The condition is self-limiting and improves in 2 to 5 years. Mast cells release histamine and cause the lesions to develop.

Factors that can aggravate chronic urticarial
1) Anti-inflammatories
2) Alcohol
3) Stress (both emotional and physical)
4) Tight clothes or heat
5) Certain foods are associated with worsening of the disorder but only in a small group of patients.

Patients with chronic urticarial might have an increased risk for autoimmune disorders including thyroid disease and diabetes.

Treatment
1) Non-sedating H1 antihistamines as first line. Certirizine 10mg daily
2) Sedating/ First generation H1 antihistamine. Hydroxyzine 25 to 50 mg daily. Diphenhydramine 25 to 50 mg daily or as needed
3) Leukotriene modifiers. Montelukast 10 mg daily. Allow one month to see results
4) Immunosuppressive drugs and phototherapy can be mobilized at specialist level.

Physical urticarias
Physical urticarias are a result of environmental stimuli.

1) **Dermatographism**. Urticarial lesions appear at the site of trauma or scratching to the skin.
   Treatment:
   a) First and second generation H1 antihistamines
   b) H2 antihistamines (Ranitidine and Cimetidine)

2) **Pressure urticarial.** Lesions appear within a day after pressure was applied to the site.
   Treatment:

Montelukast can be used to control the symptoms but treatment is often unsatisfactory.

3) **<u>Cholinergic urticarial</u>**. Small urticarial lesions form after an episode of sweating or rise in body temperature.
   Treatment:
   1) Non-sedating H1 antihistamines as first line. Certirizine 10mg daily
   2) Sedating/First generation H1 antihistamine. Hydroxyzine 25 to 50 mg daily. Diphenhydramine 25 to 50 mg daily or as needed

Other physical urticarias include:
Aquagenic urticarial – a very rare form of urticarial after contact with water
Solar urticarial – exposure to the sun. Treatment is with H1 antihistamines

Psoriasis

Psoriasis is a chronic skin condition characterized by sharply demarcated, erythematous plaques. The cause is multifactorial with a prominent genetic component. It can be triggered by various environmental factors including:

1) Stress
2) Drugs (Lithium, Beta blockers, Non steroidal anti-inflammatories, malaria medication)
3) Alcohol
4) Obesity
5) Smoking (especially pustular psoriasis)

Types of psoriasis

Plaque psoriasis

This is the most common form of psoriasis, responsible for 75-80% of cases. Single or multiple erythematous, symmetrical, scaly plaques develop with a predilection for the extensor surfaces of the knees, elbows and base of spine.

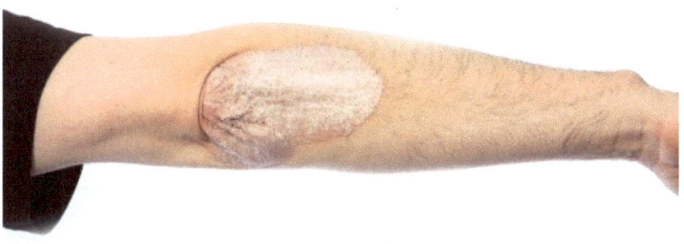

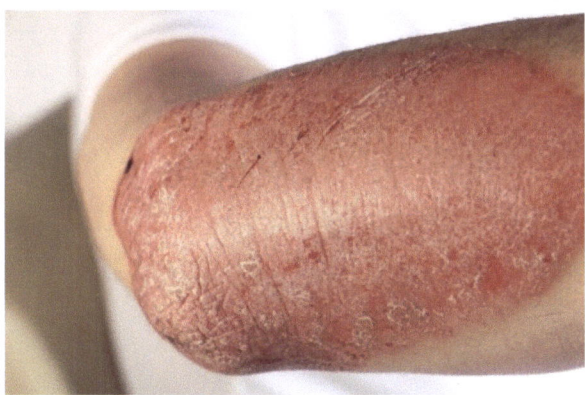

Plaque psoriasis

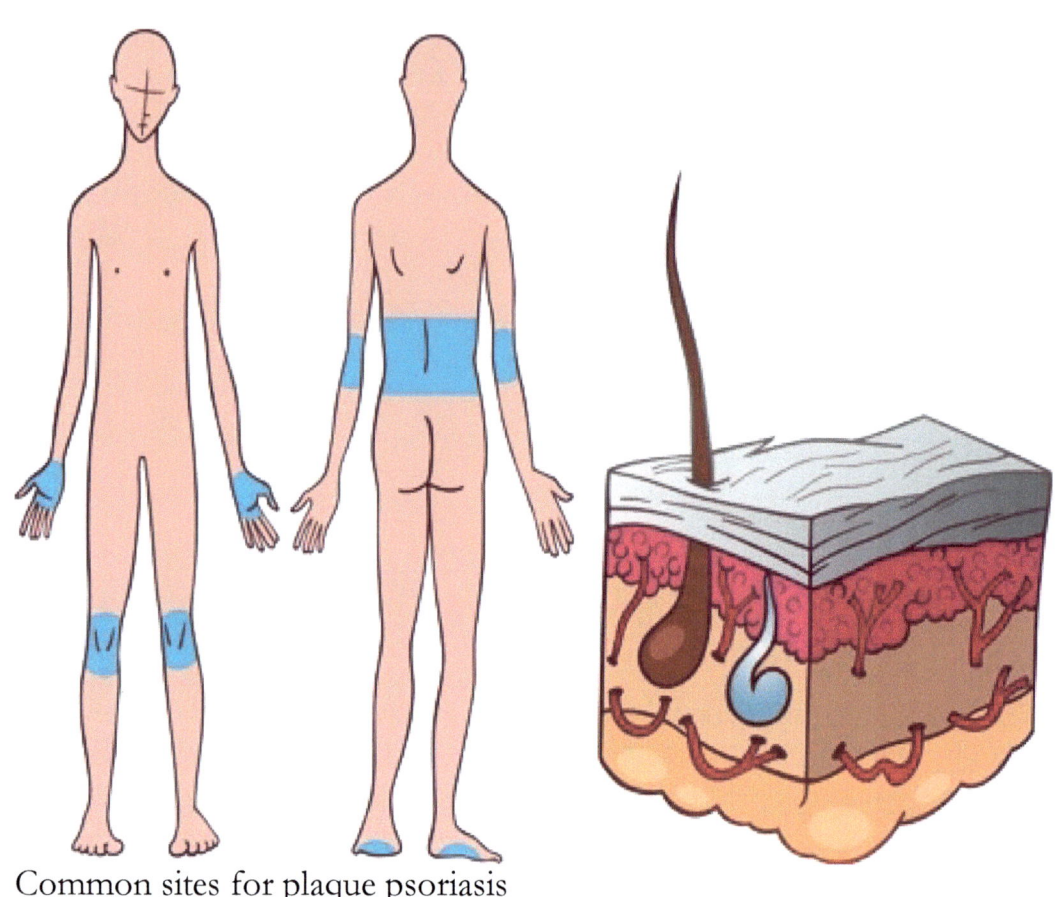

Common sites for plaque psoriasis

Flexural (Inverse) psoriasis

Lesions appear in the intertriginous areas, the groin, perineal, intergluteal, axillary and submammary folds. It is often mistaken for a fungal infection

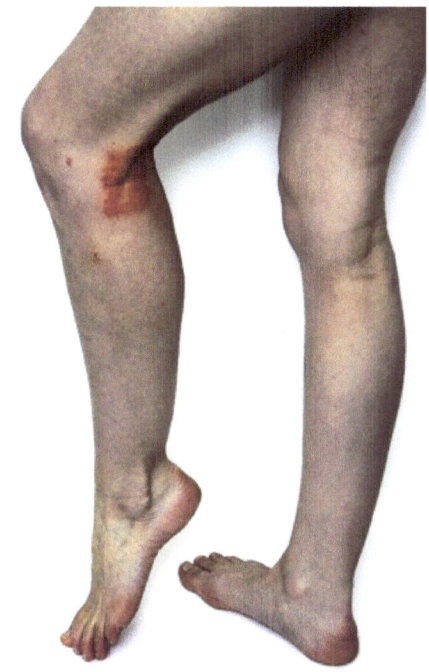

Flexural psoriasis

Pustular Psoriasis

This serious condition develops either in an existing psoriasis patient or independently and is marked by pustules with high fever. The patient can become toxic. Eruptions can occur suddenly and become life threatening.

Treatments:

Patients should be treated on a specialist level and drugs such as cyclosporine, methotrexate, infliximab and acitretin are used. Topical therapies such as vitamin D analogues, corticosteroids and calcineurin inhibitors are used as adjuvant treatment.

Guttate psoriasis

This form of psoriasis often follows an infection, most commonly streptococcal pharyngitis. The lesions are small erythematous plaques usually less than 10mm and can be misdiagnosed as pityriasis rosea. Pityriasis rosea have a more characteristic distribution and the lesions are more oval.

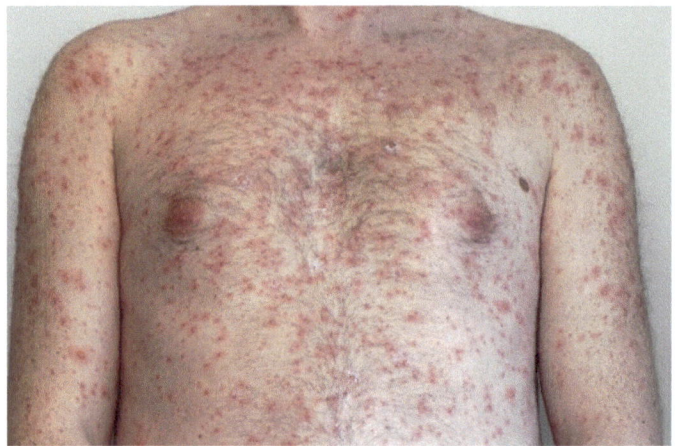

Guttate psoriasis

Erythrodermic psoriasis

In this serious form of psoriasis, the skin of the whole body becomes erythematous and scaly, leading to head and fluid loss. Inpatient care under the supervision of a Dermatologist is critical.

Nail changes associated with psoriasis:
    a. Pitting
    b. Onycholysis (nail separation from the nail bed)
    c. Leuconychia
    d. Subungual hyperkeratosis

Treatment of psoriasis

1) Topical corticosteroid creams and ointments depending on the extend of disease:
    a. Low potency for the face e.g Hydrocortisone 1%
    b. Potent steroids for the scalp -clobetasol solution or foam
    c. Potent steroids for plaques on elbows and knees - clobetasol or betamethasone 0.05%
2) Vitamin D analogue, calcipotriol – suppress proliferation of keratinocytes. Due to the side effect of inducing hypercalcemia, the maximum limit for use is 100g per week in adults, 75g per week for children over 12 and 50g per week in children aged 6-12.
3) Calcipotriol and corticosteroid combinations
4) Topical retinoid e.g tazarotene 0.05% once a day to plaques
5) Calcineurin inhibitors - primecrolimus 1% and tacrolimus 0.1%
6) Methotrexate 10 to 25mg per mouth/subcutaneous/ intramuscular per week
7) Cyclosporine 2.5mg/kg per day, supervised by a specialist Dermatologist
8) Biologic immune modifying agents – infliximab, ustekinumab on specialist level
9) Tar has fallen out of favour due to newer, more patient-friendly preparations
10) UV light – Treatment with UVB radiation is effective. It can be in the form of narrow band UVB or Psoralen UVA.

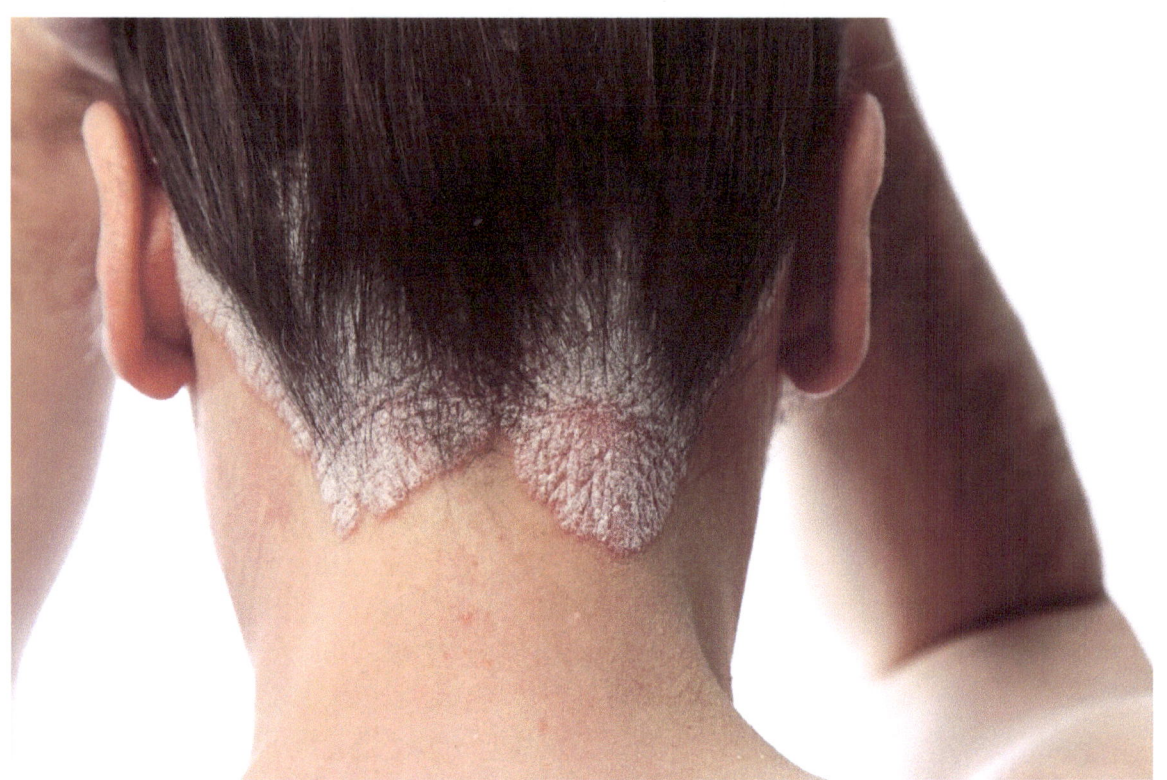

Psoriasis affecting the scalp

Papules, nodules and benign neoplasms

Molluscum contagiosum

This is a common lesion caused by the poxvirus. Lesions are pearly shaped with a central umbilicus. They can be solitary or grouped and tend to resolve spontaneously. It is more common in children. In adults it's often spread by contact sports or sexual contact. Severe outbreaks can occur in the setting of immunosuppression. Scratching, breaking or touching the lesions can cause spread. It can be seen anywhere on the body except on the palms and soles.

Treatment
It is a self-limiting condition and should be left to resolve spontaneously.
In problematic lesions, the following treatments can be used:
1) Curettage and cryotherapy
2) Cantharidin can be used to treat the lesions topically.
3) Salicylic acid
4) Topical retinoids e.g adapalene or tazoratene
5) Oral cimetidine

Warts

Warts are benign epidermal neoplasms. The human papilloma virus group is responsible for their formation. Plantar and common warts are due to HPV 1,2,3,4 and 27. Genital warts are cause by HPV 6 and 11.
Warts are spread by simple contact of the skin and can be contracted from moist surfaces of communal pools and saunas.

Common warts (Verruca vulgaris)

These lesions can be found on any part of the body but is most commonly seen on the hands. They are cauliflower-like, dome shaped lesions. Black dots will appear when the capillaries become thrombosed.

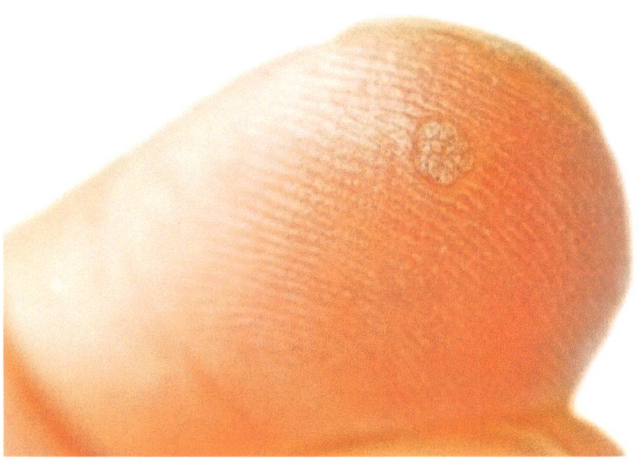

Treatment

1) Salicylic acid
2) Liquid nitrogen cryotherapy. Freeze time should be 10 seconds and repeated in 2 to 4 weeks.
3) Electrocautery

Plantar warts

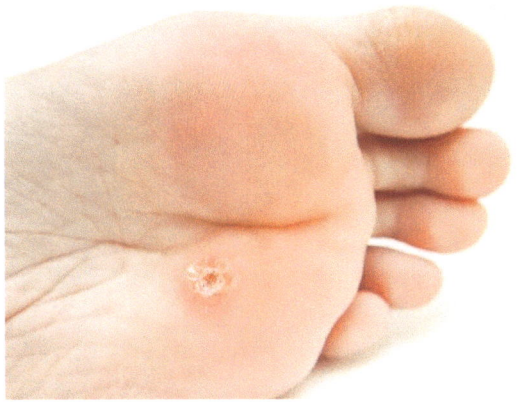

They can be single, scattered over the foot or grouped together producing an area of thick skin.

Treatment:
1) Debride the wart every 2-3 weeks
2) Salicylic acid
3) Cryotherapy with liquid nitrogen
4) 5-fluorouracil cream once to twice a day for 3 months
5) Soaking for 30 minutes daily in Formalin 4% solution

Flat warts (Verruca plana)

These warts usually occur on the dorsum of the hands and face and can be light brown to pink papules. They are flat topped and can spread by means of scratching and shaving.

Treatment
1) Imiquimod cream 5 days a week for 3 to 4 months
2) Cryotherapy
3) 5-Fluorouracil cream twice a day for a month

Periungual warts

Warts around the area of the nail are very resistant to treatment and can be partially protected by the nail against physical treatments.

Treatment
1) Cryotherapy can be attempted but is not very effective
2) Keratolytics e.g salicylic acid and lactic acid

3) Excision of the wart
4) Duct tape occlusion. Apply duct tape for 6 days without removing it. Open the wart for 12 hours and repeat.

Dermatofibroma

These are collections of fibrous tissue and blood vessels, more commonly seen in women and on the lower limbs. It is often as a result of trauma, insect bites or local infections. Clinically it's a round, firm nodule with a darker edge. It's rarely larger than 10mm.

Treatment

Surgical excision for cosmetic purposes but this can lead to more unsightly scars.

Epidermal cysts (sebaceous cysts)

These keratin-forming cysts most often appear on the back, chest, face and behind the ears. They have an opening to the surface and can discharge keratin to the outside but can also leak keratin into the dermal layer. This will cause a severe inflammatory reaction.

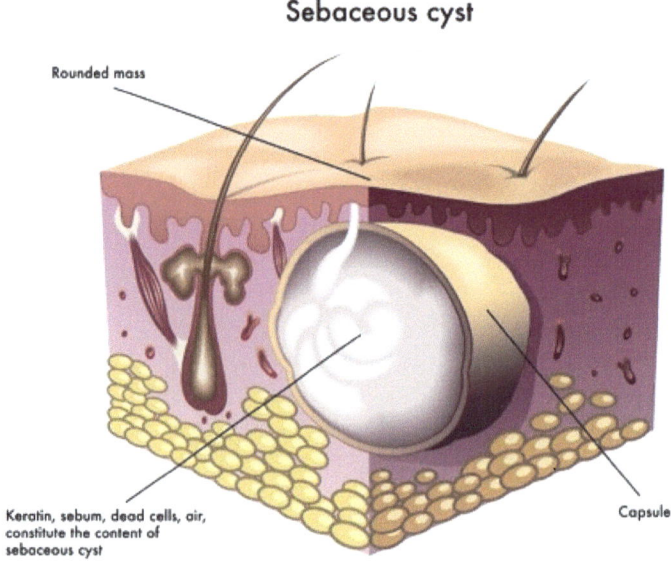

Sebaceous cyst

Rounded mass

Keratin, sebum, dead cells, air, constitute the content of sebaceous cyst

Capsule

Treatment

Excision is the treatment of choice

Milia

Milia are small, white keratin cysts that are most often seen around the eyes and the cheeks.

Treatment
Puncture of the lesions with a needle or pin

Pyogenic granuloma

Pyogenic granulomas are benign vascular lesions due to an inflammatory process. They are dome-shaped, often with a narrowing around the base, bleeds profuse when injured and usually has a moist surface.

Treatment
Pyogenic granulomas require surgical excision or curettage. Electrocautery is useful to control bleeding.

Keratoacanthoma

This benign lesion was previously considered malignant due to the histological similarities to squamous cell cancers. They are dome shaped and have a central crater filled with keratin. They grow very rapidly and can resolve spontaneously. UV radiation, Fitzpatrick I, II and II and trauma can make an individual more prone to develop these lesions.

Treatment
Surgical excision is the treatment of choice.

Skin tags

Skin tags are common on the neck and axillae of many people. Obesity and advancing age will make a person more predisposed for these benign lesions.

Treatment
1) Snip excision

2) Cautery
3) Cryotherapy

Pilomatricoma

This benign tumor of the hair follicle is often seen on the face of children and can enlarge up to 4cm. Treatment is simple excision.

Lipoma

Lipomas are benign fat cell tumours presenting as firm nodules. They can be familial or sporadic and is treated by excision of the entire lump.

Lichen planus

Lichen planus is a disorder with an unknown ethiology. Middle-aged adults are most commonly affected and sites of predilection include the oral cavity, scalp, genitalia, wrists and ankles.

Clinical features: (6 P's)
1) Purple (violaceous)
2) Polygonal
3) Plaque or
4) Papule
5) Palpable
6) Pruritic

It can contain a fine network of lines called Wichenhan's striae and oral lesions may show as reticulate streaks.

Treatment
1) Topical steroids. High potency to superpotency steroids (Betamethasone diproprionate 0.5%) twice a day and mid- to low potency creams on the face.
2) Intralesional steroids e.g triamcinolone.
3) Systemic treatment – oral glucocorticoid therapy of 30 to 60mg per day for 4 to 6 weeks.

4) Phototherapy and acitretin oral retinoid at specialist level.

Non-melanoma skin cancers

Basal cell carcinoma

Basal cell carcinoma is the most common malignant skin tumors. It is locally invasive but rarely metastasize. It forms in the basal layer of the skin's epidermis and can cause destruction of all nearby structures, including bone.

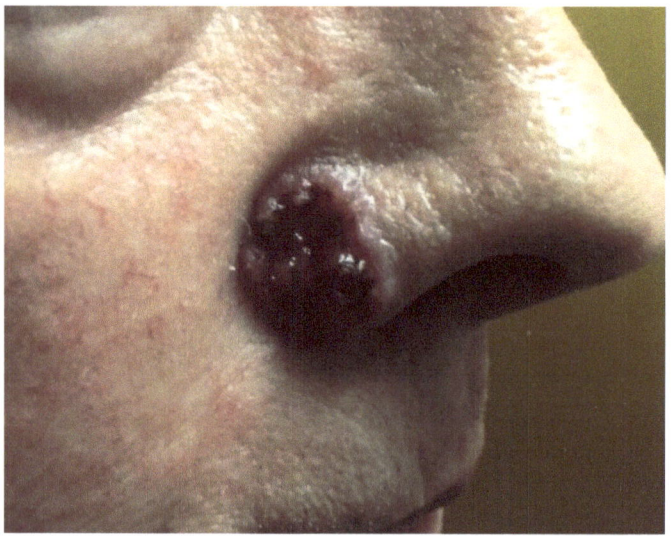

Risk factors
1) UV radiation. Childhood exposure to UV radiation can make an adult more prone to develop basal cell carcinoma. Tanning beds will increase an individual's risk to develop basal cell carcinoma
2) Immunosuppression
3) Genetic variants (Gorlin Syndrome)
4) Arsenic exposure through drinking water or medication
5) Ionizing radiation

Variants
Nodular basal cell carcinoma
These compromise the majority of basal cell carcinomas.

Clinical features:
1) Mostly on sun exposed surfaces
2) Dome-shaped nodules
3) Rolled, pearly edge with central ulceration often
4) Telangiectasia

Superficial basal cell carcinoma
This variant of basal cell carcinoma can grow horizontally for many years, forming big lesions without a nodular appearance. It is the least aggressive form of basal cell carcinomas.

Clinical features:
1) Macules, patches or plaques
2) Erythematous
3) Sometimes an atrophic center

Morphoeic
These lesions are smooth, pale white coloured patches or plaques and can have a scar-like or scleroderma appearance. The borders are undefined and local invasion is common.

Treatment
1) Surgical excision
2) Mohs microsurgery – histological evaluation of the lesion during surgery to minimize the amount of disease-free tissue that is excised
3) Electrodesiccation and curettage
4) Cryosurgery
5) Imiquimod
6) 5-Fluorouracil
7) Radiation therapy
8) Photodynamic surgery

Squamous cell carcinoma

Squamous cell carcinoma is a cancer of the epithelium of the skin. It is both locally invasive and potentially metastatic and typically affects middle-aged and elderly people. It can develop on any part of the skin's surface. Squamous cell carcinoma can originate from various lesions including:

1) Bowen's disease
2) Leukoplakia
3) Lichen sclerosis
4) Chronic infection sites
5) Actinic keratosis

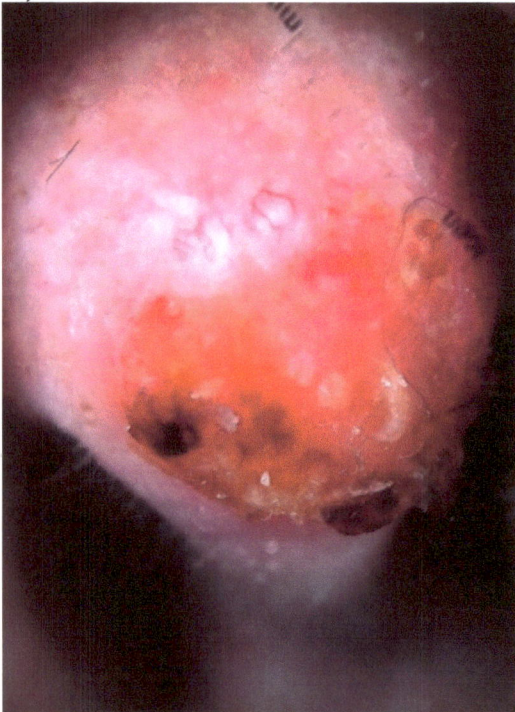

Squamous cell carcinoma

Risk factors for the development of squamous cell carcinoma include:
1) UV radiation/ Sun exposure
2) Ionizing radiation
3) Arsenic exposure
4) Human papilloma virus 6 and 11
5) People with a fair skin

Clinical features
1) Most commonly on sun exposed areas: Head, neck, hands, arms, legs, shoulders and chest.
2) Scaly patches
3) Keratotic lumps
4) Ulcers
5) Nodular lesion

Treatment
1) Excision of lesions
2) Mohs micrographic surgery
3) Radiation therapy
4) Yearly follow up with complete skin examination

Actinic keratosis has malignant potential to develop into squamous cell carcinoma and indicates that the epithelium is already dysplastic. They are red and scaly patches, sometimes easier felt than seen.

Treatment
1) Cryotherapy for individual or multiple lesions
2) Imiquimod
3) "Field treatment" is achieved when multiple lesions are present:
    a. 5-fluorouracil
    b. Ingenol mebutate
    c. Topical diclofenac 3%
    d. Retinoids (adapalene)
    e. Chemical peels

Hyperpigmented lesions

Melanocytic nevi - congenital and acquired

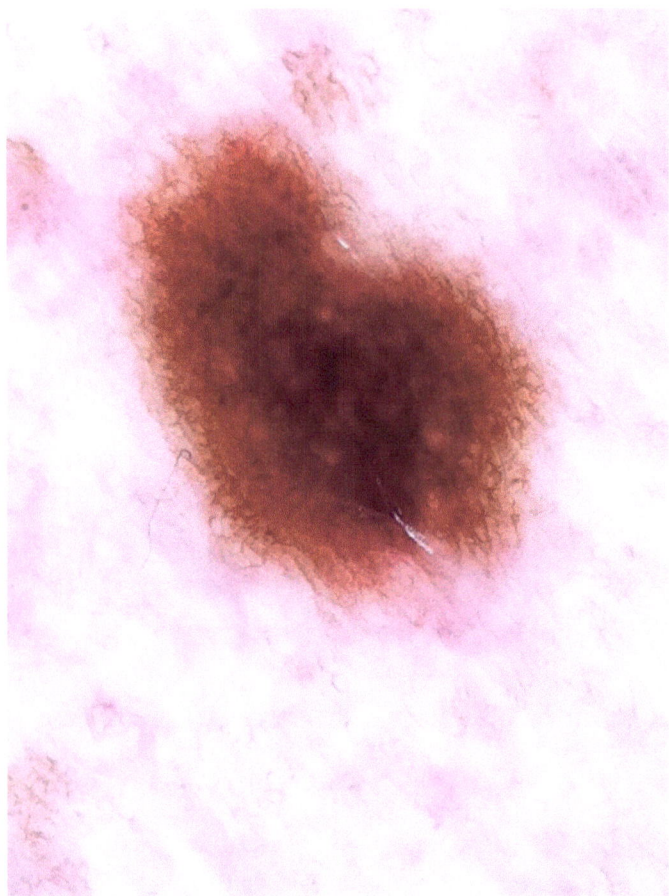

Melanocytic nevus

Melanocytic nevi are lesions of extreme importance in the primary care setting. Countless of patients will present asking you to "check their moles" and anxiety levels will soar if you are unable to recognize the features of a benign versus a malignant lesion.

Melanocytic nevi will be present on almost every human and their increase in number can be associated with sun exposure. They have a very low potential to become malignant except for atypical nevi and large congenital nevi.

Nevus cells form groups (nests) and multiply at the dermoepidermal junction. Some cells can migrate vertically into the dermis (compound nevi) or become intradermal when all the cells are within the dermis.

Melanocytic nevi remain uniform in colour, shape and size. It may contain various shades of brown or black but always has a uniformly distributed appearance. Melanomas can look similar in their early stages.

Nevi can be congenital or acquired. Acquired nevi develop after the age of 6 months and are most often seen on the areas of the skin with the most sun exposure.

Acquired nevi are classified according to their location in the skin:
1) **Junctional nevi** – situated at the dermoepidermal junction
2) **Compound nevi** – dermoepidermal and upper dermis
3) **Dermal nevi** – cells are in the dermis

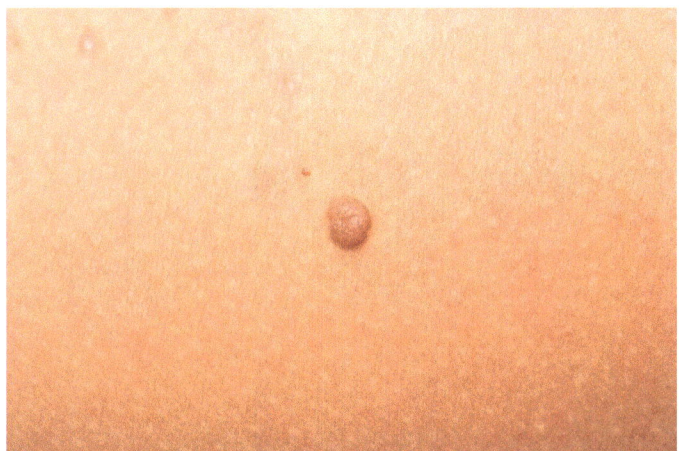

Dermal nevus

Junctional nevi are flat, compound nevi are dome shaped elevations and dermal nevi can be dome shaped, warty (verrucoid), sessile or have a stalk (pedunculated).

Treatment

Any pigmented lesion that is suspicious should be biopsied and sent for pathology. Excision of the lesion is preferred to shave biopsy.

Congenital melanocytic nevi:

These lesions are present in 1% of children and can be as large as a few centimeters in diameter. Congenital melanocytic nevi are more at risk for developing melanoma than acquired nevi. They can cover large areas of the trunk "bathing trunk" nevus, face and extremities. They are often covered with coarse hair and are uniformly pigmented.

The larger the congenital nevus, the higher risk it has for malignant transformation.

Treatment
Prophylactic removal based on each individual case. Thicker, larger nevi are most commonly removed for prevention of melanoma.

Becker's nevus

These lesions do not consist of nevus cells but are hamartomas. They present as patches of terminal hair or pigmented macules. These lesions do not contain any malignant potential and have a male to female ratio of 5 to 1.

Treatment
Treatment is for cosmetic reasons only and laser (often Q-switched ruby laser) or fractional resurfacing can be used.

Spitz nevus

These are more often seen in children and closely resemble melanoma, both clinically and pathologically. Spitz nevi are dome shaped and can be red to pink. The lower limbs and face are the most common sites. They appear suddenly and can grow fast, raising more concern for a malignant lesion. The diagnosis of a Spitz nevus is often only possible with histological evaluation after excision. All suspicious lesions should be excised for pathology.

Blue nevus

A Blue nevus is due to melanin producing melanocytes in the dermis.
They are often dome shaped with a uniformly distributed blue-black colour.

Treatment
Excision is warranted when the lesion changes or is difficult to differentiate from melanoma.

Mongolian spot

(Congenital Dermal Melanocytosis)

This lesion is common in most Asian babies, but also frequently seen in African, Indian and Hispanic babies. Less than 10% of Caucasian babies have Mongolian spots.
The spots are blue-grey and due to widely dispersed melanocytes in the dermis.
No treatment is needed and the most spots will be gone by the age of 10.

Seborrheic keratosis

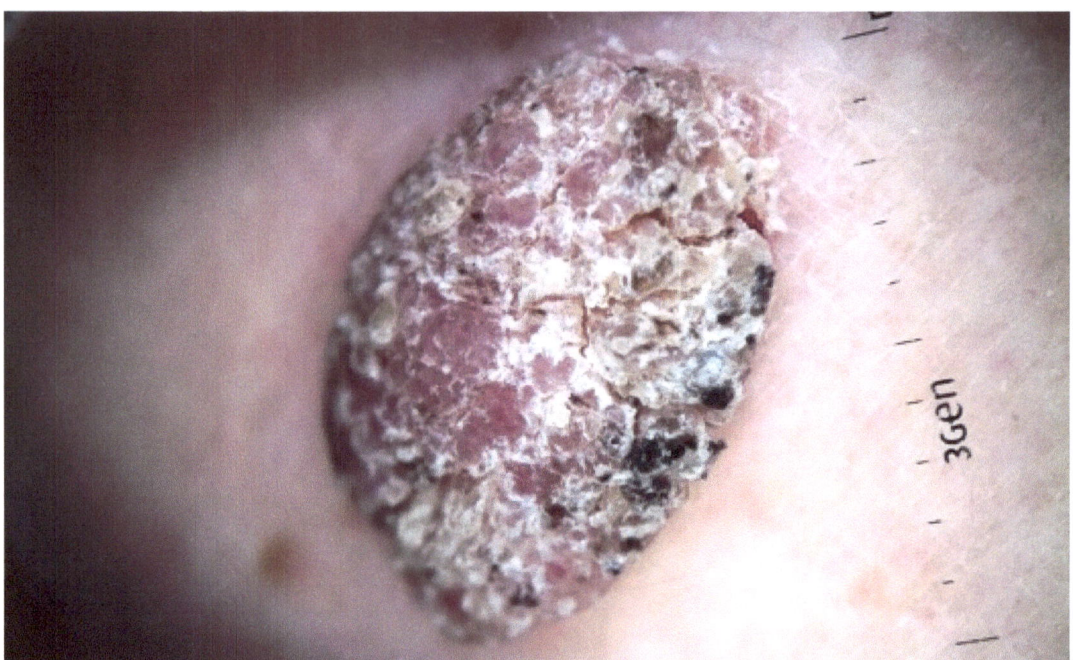

Seborrheic keratosis

These epidermal tumors are common in people over the age of 50. They can be solitary or found in large numbers in patients with a familial tendency to develop them.

They are wart-like and the classical "stuck on" description is used as a distinctive feature.

They do not have malignant potential and removing them are purely for cosmetic purposes.

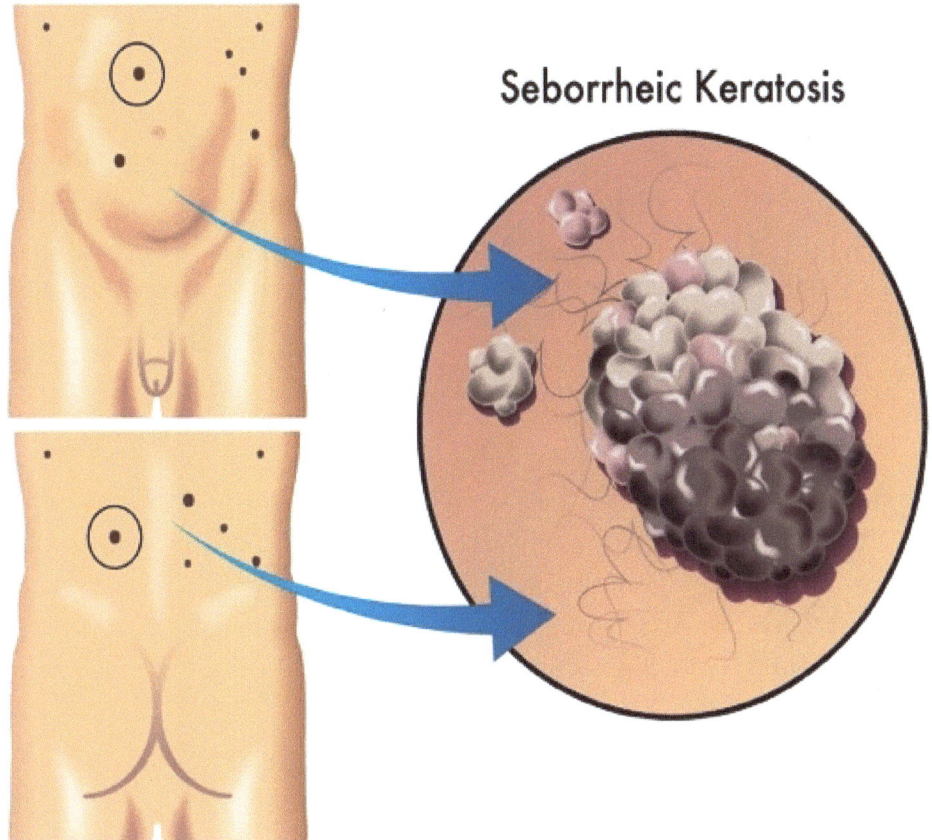

Seborrheic Keratosis

Treatment
1) Liquid nitrogen
2) Shave biopsy
3) Electrodissection.

Postinflammatory hyperpigmentation

An insult to the skin, whether it is physical, chemical, infectious or inflammatory, can cause hypermelanosis. The diagnosis is clinical.

Treatment
1) Hydroquinone
2) Retinoid creams
3) Laser treatments and chemical peels.

Melasma

Melasma is a hyperpigmentation condition that affects the face and is more common in women. It is often found in people with a darker complexion and can become more prominent during pregnancy. Contributing factors include UV radiation, darker complexions, hormones, familial tendency, and thyroid disease. The colour of the melasma depends on the level of the melanin in the skin. The deeper the melanin in the skin, the darker the melasma lesion appears.

Treatment

Treatment of melasma is difficult and unsatisfactory. Lightening creams such as hydroquinone can be used but daily application for more than 6 months might be needed. Common lightening agents include hydroquinone 4%, azelaic acid 20% cream and topical retinoids. A combination of hydroquinone 4%, flucinolone 0.01% and tretinoin 0.05% cream is often used. Chemical peels can also be applied.
Sun avoidance is crucial

Solar lentigines

These lesions are due to chronic exposure to the sun. Normal melanocytes proliferate and form these lesions in people with fair skin.

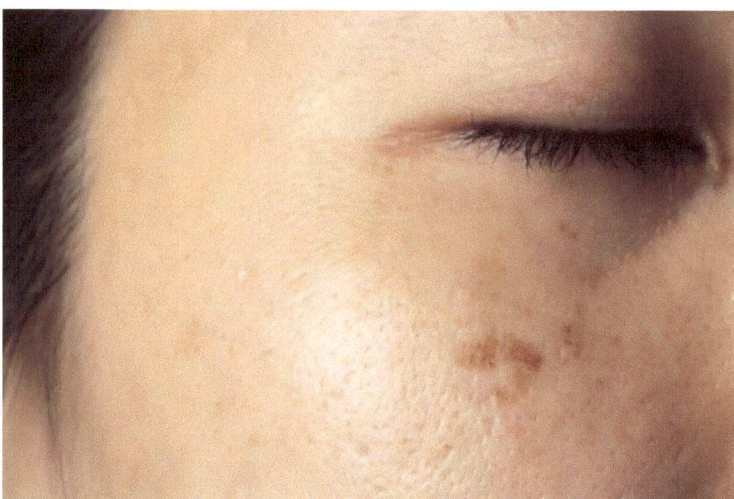

Solar lentigines

Treatment

Liquid nitrogen, applied with a short exposure time can be helpful in eliminating these lesions. Hydroquinine cream 4% is a safe alternative to lighten these marks.

Café au lait spots

These pigmented lesions often appear after sun exposure and has the appearance of flat, pigmented macules. They range from tiny macules to patches of close to 20cm. They are associated with Neurofibromatosis type 1 and McCune-Albright syndrome.

Treatment is for cosmetic reasons only and due to the association with systemic conditions, the lesions often recur.

Malignant melanoma

Malignant melanoma is the most serious form of skin cancer with a global increase in incidence rate. Caucasian people have a higher risk (10 times more) of developing melanoma compared to Black, Hispanic and Asians but a similar risk as Black people for plantar melanoma.

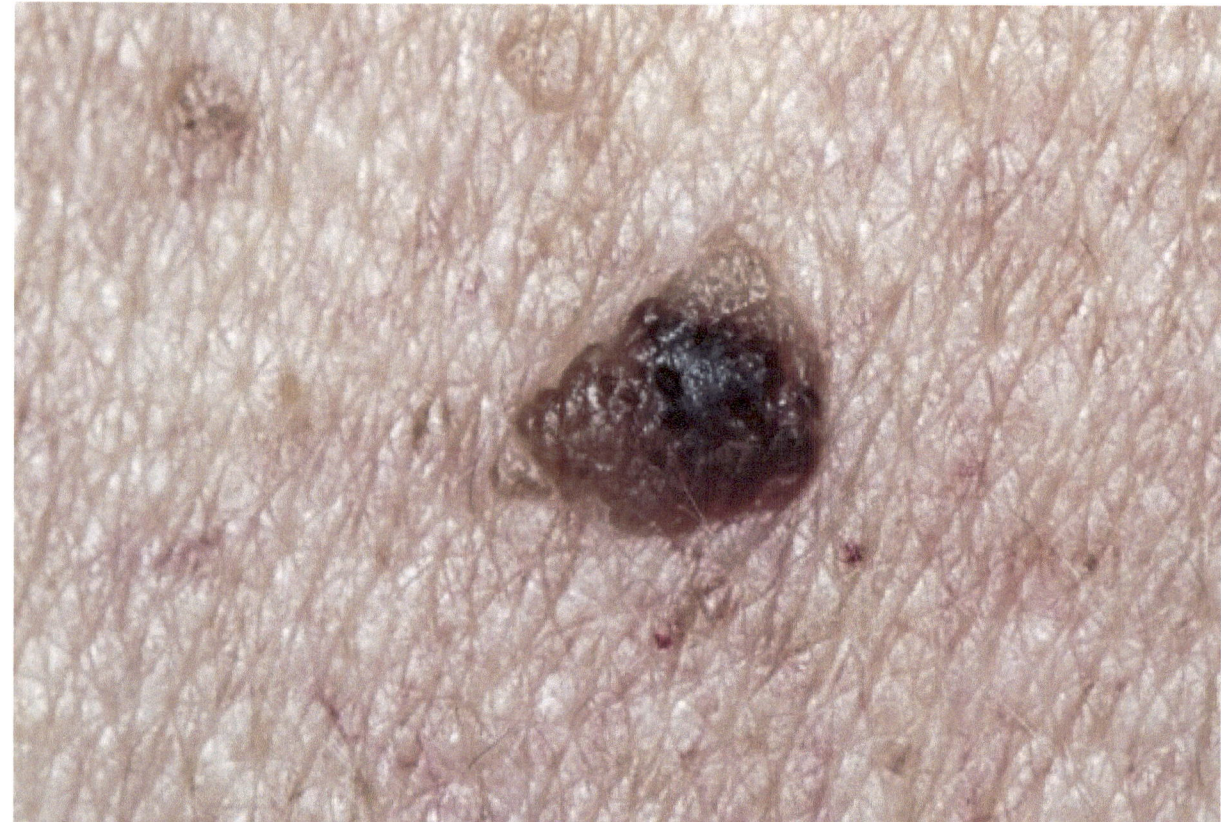

Melanoma lesion

Pathophysiology

At the time of embryogenesis, neural crest derived melanocytes migrate to the basal layer of the epidermis. Their dendritic processes then transfer melanosomes to keratinocytes. Melanosomes distribute melanin that protects DNA from UV rays. Melanin acts as a physical barrier that scatters UV rays as well as a filter that absorbs the UV rays.

Malignant melanoma develops due to the transformation and uncontrolled multiplication of melanocytes.

Risk factors

1) **Sun exposure** – UVA and UVB light. This includes artificial UV (sunbeds).
2) **Genetics** – First degree relative with melanoma, Fitzpatrick skin types 1 and 2, numerous nevi and atypical nevi
3) **Immunosupression** – Organ transplant patients, cancer patients and AIDS patients can have an impaired immune system incapable of detecting and destruction of neoplastic melanocytes.

Four clinical-histopathological subtypes

Superficial Spreading Malignant Melanoma

This type of melanoma usually forms from a more immature group of cells and aggressively grows, leading to inflammation and vascular formation. The cells grow radially in a horizontal growth phase for months to more than 10 years. Nodules appear when the lesion reaches around 2.5cm in diameter. This type comprises the majority of melanoma cases and lesions are usually located on the trunk in men and the legs in women. Due to the spreading and regression nature of the lesion, the borders become irregular and asymmetrical and can evolve into black, blue, white and red colours.

Nodular Melanoma

Poorly differentiated cells will grow without limits and produce a nodule. They represent less than 10% of melanomas and can be pedunculated, polypoid or dome shaped. Colours vary between dark brown, red-brown, red-black or can be amelanotic resembling flesh coloured dermal nevi, basal cell carcinoma, seborrheic keratosis or dermatofibroma.

Lentigo Maligna Melanoma

In well-differentiated melanocytes, the cells can remain in the epidermis and may undergo slow horizontal growth. It will be kept restrained in certain areas by a competent immune system and years of growth by such melanocytes produce Lentigo Maligna Melanoma (LMM). LMM is mostly located on the face but can occur on the arms, legs and other sun exposed sites. The radial growth phase can last for years and never develop a vertical growth phase. This is called Lentigo Maligna. In the minority of cases, the growth turns vertical and Lentigo Maligna Melanoma develops. Patients are generally over 65 years of age. The lesion is brown to black and can contain raised blue-black nodules. Nodules often only form when the lesion is 5 to 7 cm at least. Due to the long period of migration and regression, these lesions can have shapes more bizarre than Superficial Spreading Melanoma but often has a more uniform colour. The prognosis of LMM remain the same as for any other malignant melanoma.

Acral-Lentiginous Melanoma

This is the most common form of melanoma in people of African and Afro-caribean descent. Less than one tenth of melanomas in white people are Acral-Lentiginous Melanomas. The sites affected are the palms, soles, mucous membranes and fingers. These lesions tend to remain flat and can be latent for years, making it a good candidate for early detection and surgical removal. Acral-Lentiginous Melanoma is very aggressive and spreads quite early. Pigmented band appearing at the proximal nailfold (Hutchingson's sign) is suggestive of this form of melanoma

Clinical Suspicion

The **ABCD** criteria can be used to macroscopically evaluate a lesion and decide whether to biopsy it.

A-Asymmetry
B-Border irregularity
C-Colour variation or change in colour
D-Diameter enlargement
E-Evolving lesion, any change in the lesion

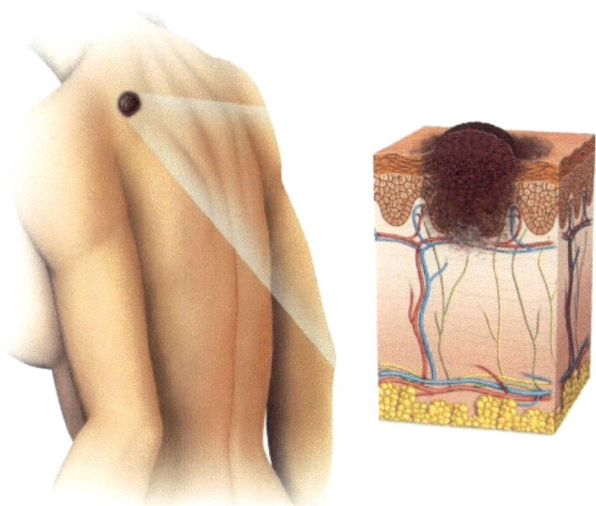

Melanoma

Management of Malignant Melanoma

Suspicious lesions should be excised. Incisional biopsies do not alter survival or promote spread and punch biopsies of the thickest area of the lesion can be performed if the suspicion for melanoma is low. Shave biopsies are not an appropriate technique for suspicious lesions.

Hypopigmented disorders

Congenital

Albinism

Albinism is a generalized hypopigmented disorder with either absent- or defective tyrosinase enzymes leading to defects in melanin production. The clinical picture is more severe in people with an absent tyrosinase enzyme and is marked by hypopigmented skin, red eyes and vision impairment. Skin cancers are frequently seen in both forms of albinism.

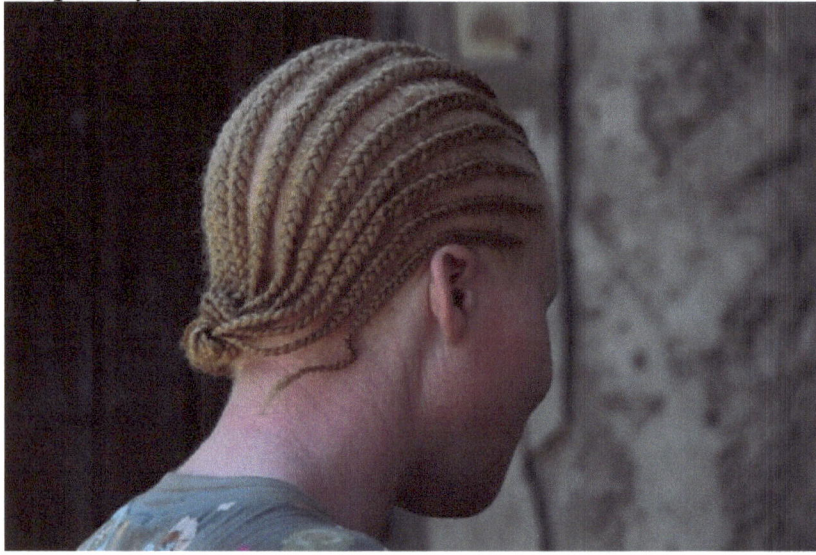

Tuberous sclerosis

Tuberous sclerosis presents with hypopigmented macules that are most commonly seen on the arms, trunk and lower limbs. Wood's lamp examination is helpful in identifying the lesions.

Phenylketonuria

The reduction of tyrosine, a precursor of melanin in patients with phenylketonuria leads to lightening of the skin and hair.

Acquired

Vitiligo

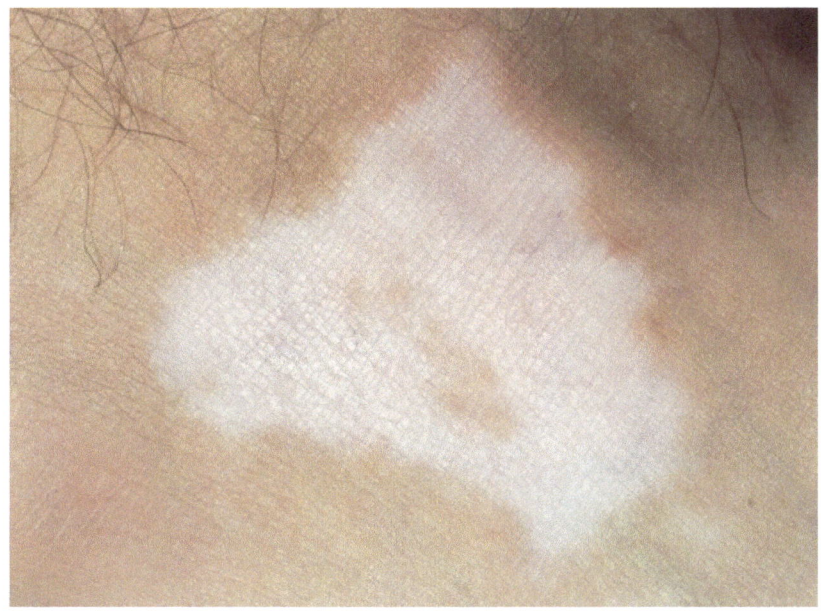

This form of acquired loss of pigmentation is still not fully understood. Histologically there is an absence of melanocytes in the epidermis with associated vitiligo antibodies at times. Vitiligo is a process of depigmentation rather than hypopigmentation. Patches are most often seen around openings of the body including the eyes, mouth, genital areas and are also often seen on the hands, axillae and body folds.

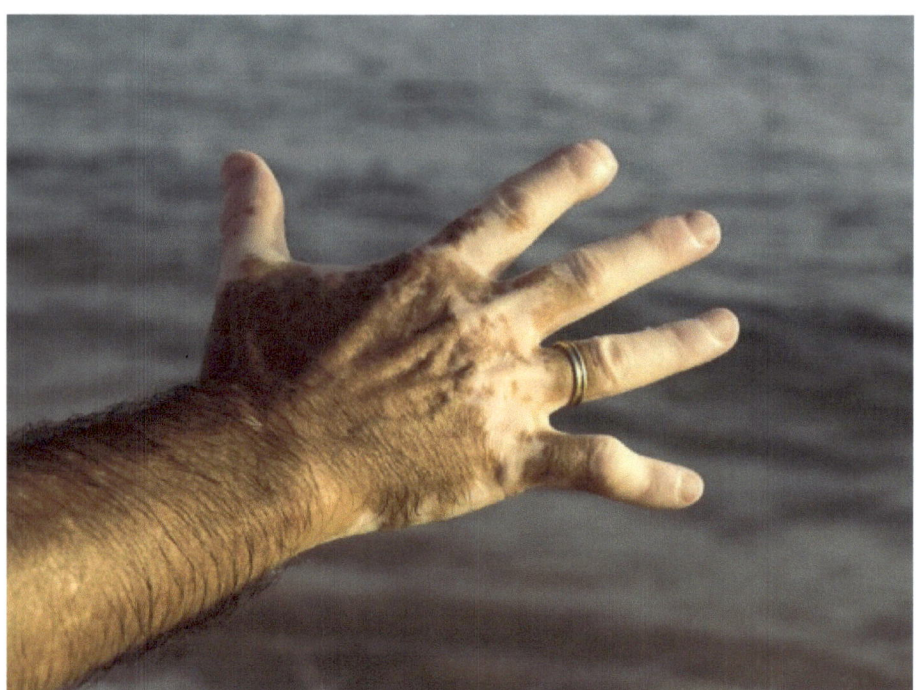

Treatment is difficult and often unsatisfactory.

Treatments:
1) Topical corticosteroids for lesions less than 10% of the total body surface and not affecting the face. Class 3 or 4 for 6 to 9 months
2) Calcineurin inhibitors. Topical calcineurin inhibitors (pimecrolimus and tacrolimus) can be used for longer periods than corticosteroid treatments.
3) Psoralen plus UV A lights and UVB light
4) Topical vitamin D analogs
5) Depigmentation of remaining pigmented skin.

Tinea versicolor

Tinea versicolor can produce hypopigmented or hyperpigmented macules. It is caused by *Malassezia* fungus

Treatment:
1) Topical antifungals: Ketoconazole 2% once a day for 2 to 3 weeks. Ciclopirox 1% twice a day for 2 weeks, Terbinafine twice a day for one to two weeks.
2) Oral treatments: Fluconazole 300mg once a week for 2 weeks. Itraconazole 200mg daily for 5 days

Ptiryasis alba

This common condition is often seen in children before the age of puberty and improves spontaneously after puberty. It affects the face, neck and arms most frequently and is characterized by scaly hypopigmented macules.

Treatment
1) Class V topical steroids
2) Calcineurin inhibitors

Idiopathic guttate hypomelanosis

These 2 to 5 mm areas of hypopigmentation on exposed areas of the skin is often associated with sun damage.
Treatment
1) Cryotherapy
2) Topical tretinoin

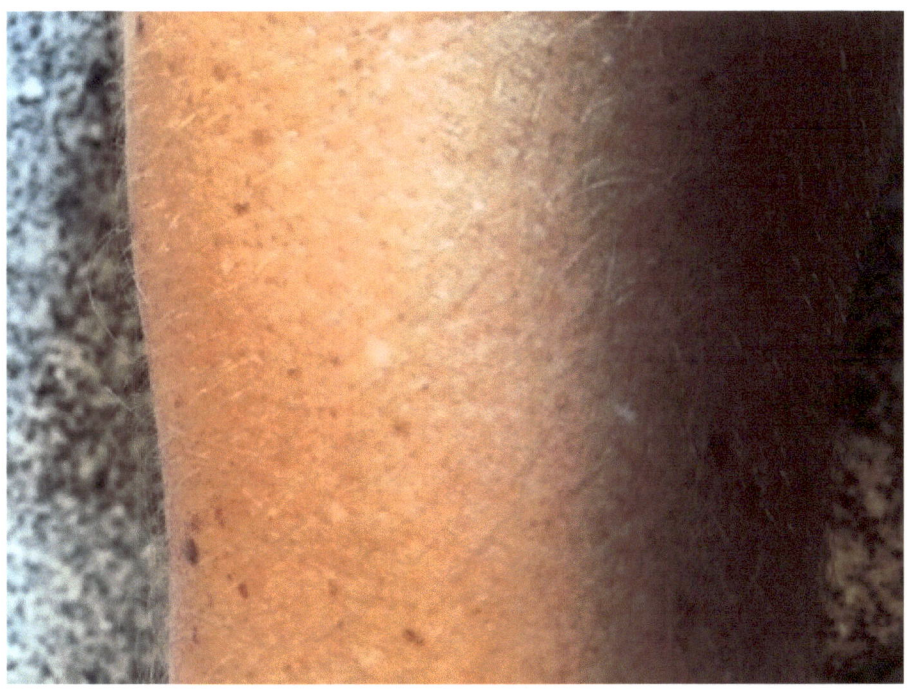

Vesicles and Bullae

Blisters are a common skin finding and can be associated with pompholyx, acute contact dermatitis, herpes simplex, herpes zoster, impetigo, burns, cold injury and insect bites.

It can be classified as **genetic** or **acquired**:
Genetic: Epidermolysis bullosa
Aquired: Pemphigus vulgaris, bullous pemphigoid

The clinical features of the blisters are dependent on the level of cleavage in the skin. The more superficial the cleavage (subepidermal/ suprabasilar), the more flaccid and fragile is the blister. Deeper cleavage levels form more tense blisters.

Epidermolysis bullosa:

This form of inherited blistering disorder affects infants. The patient will often have a family history of the same condition. Skin biopsies will confirm the diagnosis.
Other conditions that can mimic epidermolysis bullosa include herpes simplex gestationalis, autoimmune bullous disorders like pemphigoid and linear IgA and congenital porphyria.

Pemphigus vulgaris

Pemphigus vulgaris is a disorder of blister formation where the changes occur just above the basal layer (intraepidermal) of the skin causing flaccid blisters and erosions. Oral lesions often occur first, followed by skin lesions weeks to months later. Application of a little bit of pressure in a lateral direction results in exfoliation of the blister, known as Nikolsky's sign.
Pemphigus vulgaris can be a fatal if untreated.

Pemphigus vulgaris versus Bullous pemphigoid

Pemphigus vulgaris	Bullous pemphigoid
Nikolsky sign positive	Nikolsky sign negative
Young and elderly patients	Elderly patients
Flaccid, fragile blisters	Tense blisters with erythema
Oral mucosa commonly affected	Oral mucose mostly unaffected
No preceding pruritis	Pruritis present

Treatment of pemphigus vulgaris:
1) Systemic steroid therapy is the first line of treatment. Prednisone 1 to 1.5mg per kilogram. Dose can be tapered down based on response.
2) The following treatments can be used but should be overseen by a dermatologist
    a) Azathioprine
    b) Mycophenolate mofetil
    c) Dapsone

Bullous pemphoid

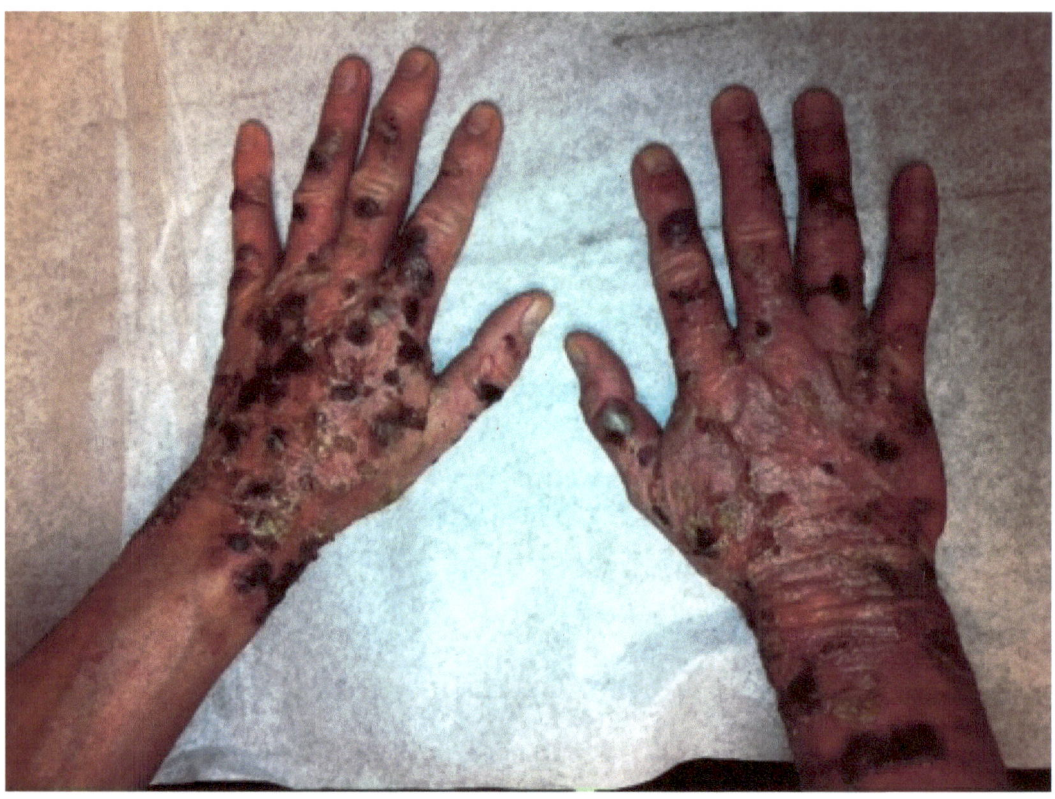

Bullous pemphigoid is an autoimmune disorder and occurs more often in the elderly. These patients have an immune response to normal tissue resulting in subepidermal blister formation.

Commonly used drugs implicated in the formation of bullous pemphigoid are:
1) Captopril
2) Ciprofloxacin
3) Clonidine
4) Enalapril
5) Furosemide
6) Ibuprofen
7) Influenze vaccine
8) Mefenamic acid
9) Nifedipine
10) Bactrim

Clinical features

24% of patients have oral lesions that are transient and mild. Bullous pemphigoid starts as an area of erythema or itchy urticarial plaques. These gradually become more edematous and also more extensive. Often patients are treated for hives for months before the diagnosis of bullous pemphigoid is made. After 1 to 3 weeks most plaques turn red or cyanotic often resembling erythema multiforme with rapidly appearing and generalized vesicles and bullae.

Sites most commonly affected:
1) Lower abdomen
2) Groin
3) Flexor surfaces of arms and legs
4) Palms and soles

Blister characteristics

1) 1 to 7 cm
2) Isolated or in clusters
3) Tense with good structural integrity
4) Nikolsky's sign negative (epidermis layer separates easily from the basal layer on exertion of sliding manual pressure)
5) Lesions rupture within 1 week leaving a rapidly healing eroded base

Course

The course of bullous pemphigoid varies from spontaneous resolution of a localized eruption to chronic relapsing generalized disease.

Treatment

The goal of treatment is to decrease the blister formation, decrease itching, promote healing and improve quality of life.

First line therapy is with corticosteroids, either topical or systemic.

Itching can be treated with hydroxyzine of 10 to 50mg every 4 hours as needed.

Topical steroids

High potency should be used (clobetasol). Topical steroids have been shown to be superior to oral steroid therapy for extensive disease.

Antibiotics

Good clinical results were obtained by using antibiotics for generalized bullous pempigoid. The antibiotics included tetracyclin, erythromycin or minocycline. These drugs seem to suppress the inflammatory response

Immunosupressive drugs

Systemic steroids are important in bullous pemphigoid treatment. It is used for patients who do not have sufficient response to topical corticosteroids, antibiotics or dapsone or who are unable to apply the topical treatments as needed. Prednisone or prednisolone at dosages of 0.5mg to 1mg per kg per day in divided dosages is used. Tapering down on therapy is recommended when the disease is under control, usually expected within 28 days. Adding dapsone to the regimen has a steroid sparing affect.

Methotrexate:

This is effective as a low dose oral pulse therapy in patients with generalized disease. Start with a dose of 10mg per week and adjust upward with 2.5mg per week until a positive response occurs. The dosage can then be decreased by 2.5mg per week every 2 months and then discontinued. Itching can be treated with clobetasol. Folic acid should be given to decrease hematological side effects.

Indications for referral:

The management of these patients is often a team effort involving a dermatologist and the primary care physician.

Referral to other specialists should be considered:

1) Ophthalmology if ocular involvement occur
2) Gastroenterology when a patient has symptoms suggestive of esophageal disease
3) Otolaryngologist when the pharynx and larynx is affected.

Herpes zoster

The term Varicella is used to describe the condition known as chickenpox, caused by the Herpes Zoster virus. A rash occurs after an incubation period of about 3 weeks, appearing macular and then developing into papules and vesicles. After recovery, the virus becomes latent and remains in the posterior root ganglia.

When the herpes virus is reactivated, a rash known as herpes zoster or "shingles" appear. The rash follows a dermatome unilaterally and most commonly in the area of T5 to L2. The rash contains many painful vesicles that crusts over before healing. Pain can remain for weeks to years after the rash disappears.

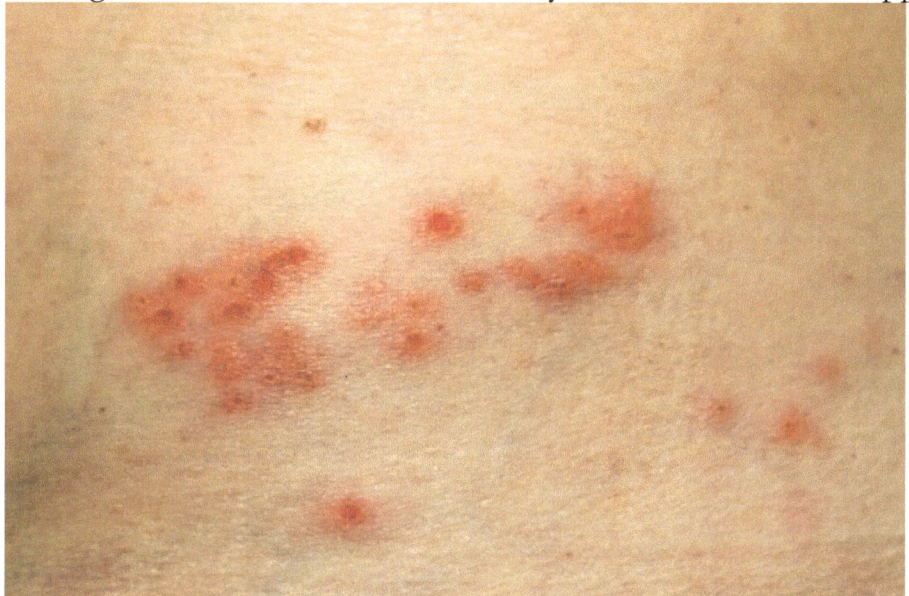

Shingles rash

Diagnosis
Serum: Varicella IgG can be identified in the serum of a person with immunity against herpes zoster.
Direct immunofluorescence: Sampling of the base of a vesicle for virology can be used to identify the virus.

Treatment
1) Acyclovir: 800mg 5 times a day for 7 to 10 days
2) Valcyclovir: 1g three times a day for 7 days
3) Famciclovir: 500mg three times a day for 7 days.

Herpes simplex

Two types of herpes viruses are responsible for herpes simplex lesions. Type 1 affecting the lips and face most commonly and type 2 affecting the genital areas. Both types can affect any area of the body.

Transmission can be from oral contact, oral-genital contact or through intercourse.

Primary infection occurs when the person contracting the virus has no antibodies against the virus (first time exposure). Symptoms usually appear within a week after contact, resulting in multiple ulcerating and crusting lesions. Systemic symptoms include fever, malaise, muscle ache and headache. Lymphadenopathy is common.

Secondary (non-primary infection) occur after the development of antibodies and is usually milder with fewer systemic symptoms.

Viral shedding can occur even when there are no active lesions.

Diagnosis

The condition is usually diagnosed clinically when there are multiple vesicles with an erythematous base.

The presence of the virus can be confirmed with viral culture, antibody testing, polymerase chain reaction (PCR) or serology type-specific testing.

Treatment

Acyclovir

Genital Herpes: Initial episode – 200mg 5 times a day for 10 days/ 400mg 3 times a day for 10 days

Non-primary episode: 200mg 5 times a day for 5 days/ 400mg 3 times a day for 5 days/ 800mg twice a day for 5 days

Oral lesions: 200 to 300 mg 5 times a day for 5 days.

Topical treatment: Genital herpes: Apply 6 times a day for 7 days

Herpes labialis: Apply 5 times a day for 3 days

Valcyclovir:

Genital herpes: Primary – 1g twice a day for 10 days

Non-primary episode: 500mg twice a day for 3 days

Cold sores: 2g twice a day for 1 day

Famciclovir:
Genital herpes: Primary episode: 250mg 3 times a day for 10 days
Non-primary: 1000mgtwice a day for 1 day.
Cold sores: 1500mg single dose.

Dermatitis herpetiformis

This gluten-sensitive enteropathy associated condition (up to 70% association) causes vesicles on the extensor surfaces of the limbs as well as the buttocks.

Linear IgA disease

This condition causes blisters much alike bullous pemphigoid. The split in the skin occurs at the subepidermal layer, causing tense blisters. The blisters tend to be grouped around the umbilicus, face and genitalia and can be seen in both children and adults.

Thermal bullae

Blisters due to thermal injury should be kept intact as long as possible. Pain can be managed by acetaminophen in minor burn blisters.

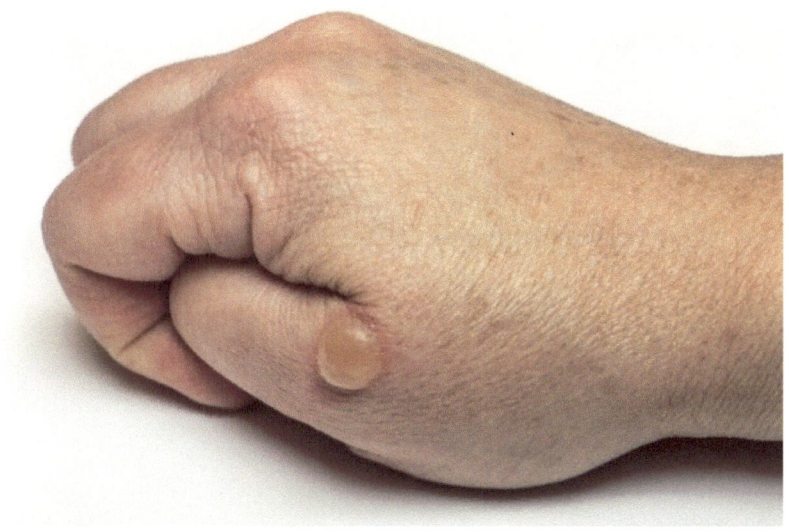

Hair disorders

Hair loss

Diffuse:

Telogen effluvium

This condition is often associated with a major stressor in the person's life, including illness, surgery, accidents, childbirth (telogen gravidarum), rapid weight loss, or emotional stress. Hair in the anagen phase are forced into the telogen phase by these stressors and cause a diffuse pattern of hair loss after about 90 days.

Diagnosis:
Hair pull test: 50-60 hairs are grasped and a quick tug will deliver more than 6 hairs in a positive test.

Treatment:
Removal or correction of the causative stressor will result in regrowth.

Systemic conditions leading to hair loss:
1) Iron deficiency
2) Thyroid disease
3) Systemic lupus erythematosus
4) Secondary syphilis
5) Alopecia totalis

Androgenic alopecia (male pattern balding)
This is due the effect of androgens on genetically susceptible people. Hair starts thinning at the anterior aspect of the scalp, the temples and the vertex, leading to bald patches in the majority of men over 70 years of age.
Treatment:
1) Minoxidil topical treatments. Foam 5% apply twice or solution 2% apply twice a day
2) Finasteride 1mg per day

Male pattern hair loss in women can be treated with the above agents as well as Spironolactone 50 to 200mg in 1 to 2 divided doses

Circumscribed

Alopecia areata

Alopecia areata, a form of non-scarring hair loss can have a chronic course. An area of discreet hair loss is often seen on the scalp but can affect any part of the body. Alopecia areata can progress into alopecia totalis (whole scalp) or alopecia universalis (whole body hair loss).

The highest prevalence of alopecia areata is during the 3rd decade of life.

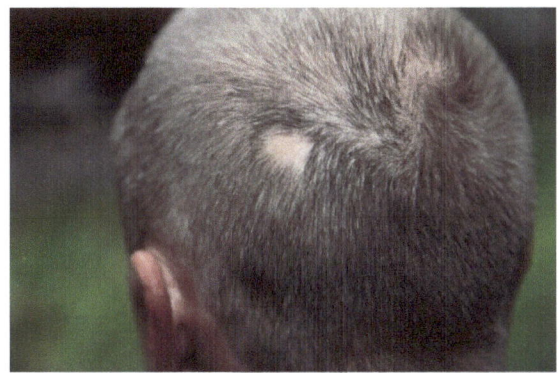

Perifollicular inflammation is thought to be the cause for this condition. The inflammation causes premature transition of the anagen follicles (active hair growth) to the catagen and telogen phases (involution and resting phases) Autoimmunity, genetics, infections, vaccinations and emotional stress have been implicated in the development of alopecia areata.

The areas of hair loss have the following characteristics:
1) Smooth skin
2) Circular patches of hair loss
3) Discreet areas with complete hair loss
4) Develops over days to weeks
5) Pruritus or burning can precede the hair loss
6) Exclamation mark hair

More than half of people with alopecia areata can have nail involvement. Features include:
1) Pitting

2) Red spots on the lunulae
3) Onycholysis
4) Trachyonychia

Treatment:
1) Intralesional corticosteroids: Triamcinolone 2.5-5mg/ml for face, eyebrows and beard. 5-10mg/ml for scalp.
2) Topical steroids (potent): Betamethasone 0.05% for 3 months
3) Topical immunotherapy (Dermatologist discretion)

Trichotillomania

This is a condition in which the person plucks hair from the scalp repeatedly, leading to atypical hair loss patters.

Traction

Certain hairstyles result in constant traction on the hair follicles and can lead to permanent hair loss. The most commonly affected areas include the frontal and temporal regions.

Hair loss with abnormal scalp:

Tinea capitis can cause inflammation of the scalp and lead to hair loss. Psoriasis is also implicated in hair loss

Conditions causing scarring
1) Discoid Lupus erythematosus
2) Lupus vulgaris
3) Lichen Planus

Hirsutism

(excessive hair growth)

Hirsutism is excessive, male pattern hair growth in females. It is usually a sign of androgen excess. Androgens interact with the hair follicles and lead to the change in hair growth.

The androgens most commonly implicated are:
1) Testosterone
2) Dehydroepiandrosterone
3) Androstenedione

Causes
1) Familial
2) Polycystic ovarian disease
3) Ovarian tumors
4) Adrenal tumors
5) Insulin resistance syndromes

Treatment:
1) Oral contraceptive
2) Spironolactone
3) Flutamide
4) Finasteride
5) Insulin lowering treatments (e.g metformin) in Insulin resistance syndromes

Hypertrichosis
Hypertrichosis is the term used when there is excessive hair growth but not following a male secondary sexual pattern.

Causes:
1) Congenital
2) Medications including minoxidil and steroids
3) Anorexia nervosa

Nail abnormalities:

Onycholysis – nail elevation due to accumulation of debris under the nail plate. 	1) Psoriasis 2) Tinea infections 3) Thyrotoxicosis
Pitting	1) Psoriasis 2) Alopecia areata 3) Sarcoidosis 4) Lichen planus
Beau's lines (Deep lines running from side to side of the nail)	Major systemic disease including 1) Syphilis 2) Zinc deficiency 3) Chemotherapy 4) Diabetes 5) Malnutrition
Yellow Nails	Yellow nail syndrome (Bronchiectasis plus pleural effusions plus lymphedema)
Loss of nail cuticle	Paronychia/ Infection

Brittle nails 	1) Iron deficiency 2) Thyroid disease
Trachyonychia (sandpapered nails)	1) Lichen planus 2) Alopecia areata 3) Psoriasis
Clubbing	1) Cyanotic heart disease 2) Lung disease – carcinoma, bronchiectasis, cystic fibrosis 3) Liver disease 4) Thyrotoxicosis 5) Inflammatory bowel disease 6) Celiac disease
White nails	1) Hypoalbuminemia/ liver disease 2) Anemia 3) Malnutrition 4) Zinc deficiency
Green-blue nails	Pseudomonas infection
Melanonychia (longitudinal brown lines) 	1) Normal is some ethnic groups 2) Pregnancy 3) Psoriasis 4) Addison disease 5) HIV infection 6) Hyperthyroidosis 7) Melanoma of the nail unit

Koilonychia (spoon shaped nails)	Iron deficiency anemia
Splinter hemorrhage	1) Trauma 2) Infective endocarditis 3) Anemia 4) Hematological malignancy 5) Vasculitis

Paronychia

When the nail fold becomes infected, it appears red and swollen. It can be bacterial or fungal in origin.
Chronic paronychia is caused by chronic inflammation of the nail fold due to breakdown of the skin's barrier through irritant and allergen exposures. Pseudomonas has been implicated in some infections.

Treatment
Acute paronychia:
1) Drain if an abscess is present
2) Mupirocin and corticosteroid combinations (betamethasone 0.05%)
3) Oral antibiotics for susceptible organisms if the disease is more widespread

Chronic paronychia
1) Avoid the irritant
2) Keep hands dry
3) Topical corticosteroids
4) Treatment with topical antifungals can assist in recovery. Chronic paronychia can become colonized with candida species that will delay healing.

Pseudomonas
1) Treatment with acetic acid or chlorine (one part chlorine, 4 parts water) two to three times a day
2) Oral treatment includes Ciprofloxacin 500mg twice a day for 4 weeks.

Onychomycosis
(See Fungal Infections Chapter)

Pregnancy related disorders

Pregnancy can aggravate or change the appearance of many existing skin conditions. It can also cause new rashes to appear.

Pruritic Urticarial Papules and Plaques of Pregnancy (PUPPP)

Also known as polymorphic eruption of pregnancy. It is a common condition with unclear origin, affecting women during the third trimester of their pregnancy. An erythematous papular and pruritic rash appear on the abdomen, usually at the site of the striae and spreads to the arms and buttocks. The lesions coalesce to form plaques and spare the face, palms and soles (unlike pemphigoid gestationalis). The rash can worsen throughout the last days of pregnancy and immediately after delivery of the baby and then spontaneously resolves. It usually does not recur in future pregnancies.

Treatment
1) Low to mid potent topical corticosteroids (triamcinolone acetate 0.1%, Betamethasone 0.05%)
2) Non-sedating antihistamines
3) Oatmeal baths

Pemphigoid gestationalis
Pemphigoid gestationalis is a blistering disorder associated with pregnancy, usually occurring during the second and third trimester and has a substantial risk of affecting the fetus. It tends to become worse in subsequent pregnancies.
The first symptom to appear is usually pruritis, followed by an urticarial rash containing papules and plaques around the umbilicus. The rash quickly evolves into blisters that ruptures and heals without scarring. Pemphigoid gestationalis does not affect mucous membranes. It can affect the fetus and lead to pemphigoid skin lesions in the newborn.
Diagnosis can be confirmed with a biopsy of the affected skin near the site of the blister and investigated by direct immunofluorescence.

Treatment

1) Mid to high potency topical corticosteroids
2) Non-sedating oral antihistamines

Prurigo of pregnancy

This relatively common condition often develops in the second or third trimester and presents as erythematous nodules on the extensor surfaces of the arms and trunk. It has an excoriated appearance due to the intense pruritus. The etiology remains unclear.

Treatment

1) Low to mid potency topical corticosteroids
2) Non-sedating oral antihistamines

Severe generalized pruritis:

This can occur due to a condition called intrahepatic cholestasis of pregnancy. Women who have generalized pruritus should be investigated by means of serum bile acid levels and aminotransferases. A suspicion of intrahepatic cholestasis of pregnancy should prompt a referral to Obstetrics.

Light induced skin disorders

Sunburn

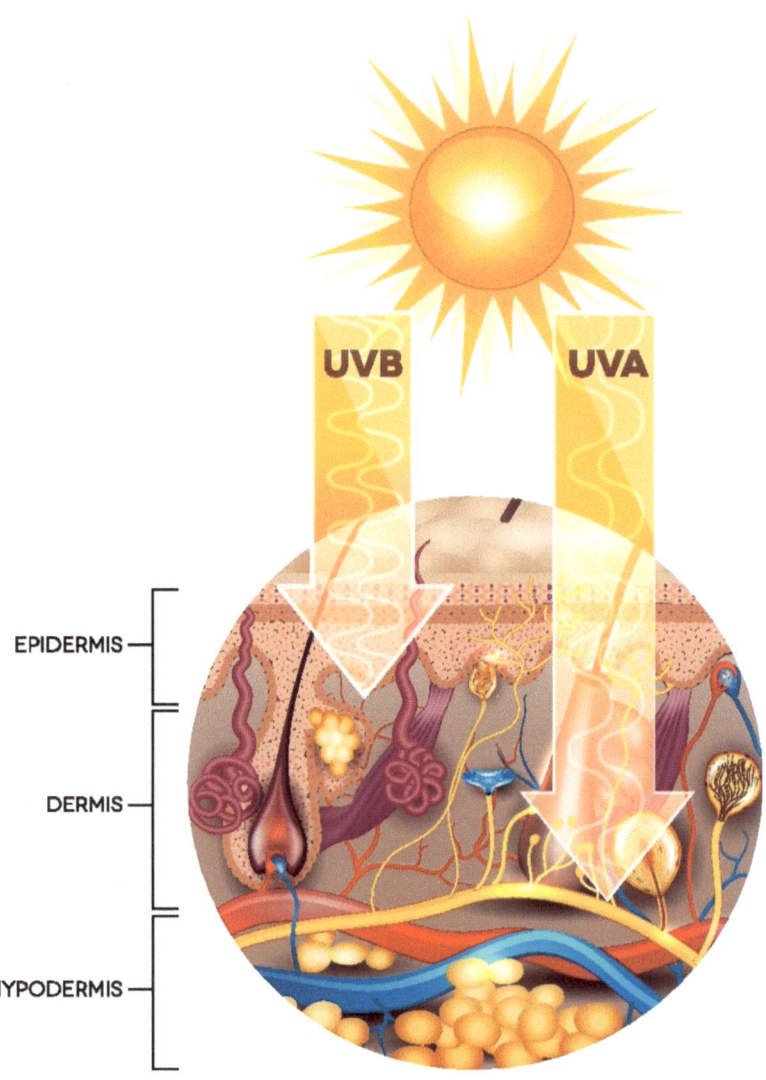

Sun avoidance and sun protection is the only efficient way to prevent the discomfort from sunburn. Once the skin is burnt, very little will ease the symptoms.

Treatment
1) Calamine lotion
2) Ibuprofen for discomfort

Polymorphic light eruption

This is an idiopathic photodermatosis and is often referred to as a "sun allergy". Women are more affected and it can start as young as adolescence.
The rash ranges from papules to plaques and blisters appear on the sun-exposed areas of the skin. The amount of light needed is very individual but patients can tolerate a certain minimum light before the rash appears. Polymorphic light eruption rashes are not seen in people who are exposed to sunlight throughout the year.

Treatment
1) Phototherapy
2) Anti-malarials - hydroxychloroquine
3) Beta-carotene with limited results.

A variant of Polymorphic light eruption is **Juvenile spring eruption**, a condition found in young boys and presents with blisters on the face, ears and hands.

Chronic actinic dermatitis

This condition presents as eczema that affects the sun exposed areas of the skin.
Photocontact allergies are frequent in these cases and most often it is due to photoallergens in sunscreens.

Actinic prurigo

This condition usually occurs in childhood but can be present at infancy. It can run in families and is more commonly seen in people with a Native American ancestry.

Clinical features

1) Pruritus
2) An eczematous rash develops on the face and hands
3) Papules and nodules

Treatment:

1) Sun protection
2) Phototherapy
3) Topical corticosteroids

STEROID POTENCY TABLE

SUPER HIGH POTENCY - GROUP 1	CLOBETASOL PROPRIONATE
HIGH POTENCY – GROUP 2 AND 3	BETHAMETHASONE DIPROPRIONATE 0.05% FLUCINONIDE 0.05% BETHAMETHASONE VALERATE 0.1%
MEDIUM POTENCY – GROUP 4	TRIAMCINOLONE ACETONIDE 0.1% MOMETASONE FUROATE 0.1%
LOWER – MID POTENCY – GROUP 5	FLUOCINOLONE ACETONIDE 0.025%
LOW POTENCY - GROUP 6	FLUOCINOLONE ACETONIDE 0.01%
LEAST POTENT – GROUP 7	HYDROCORTISONE 1%

www.ingramcontent.com/pod-product-compliance
Lightning Source LLC
Chambersburg PA
CBHW050725180526
45159CB00003B/1135